LIFE AFTER
WEIGHT LOSS
SURGERY

JOHN SIMONE

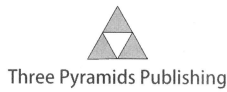

Three Pyramids Publishing

Life After Weight Loss Surgery

Three Pyramids Publishing
PO Box 432
Pine Plains, NY 12567-0432 USA

Manufactured in the United States of America.

First Edition, October 2010

ISBN-10: 1-886289-00-X
ISBN-13: 978-1-886289-00-0

Book design, typesetting and editing by John Simone

Illustrations by Carol Versace

Cover art by gnibel.com

Photographs of the author (cover and "after" photos) by Joe Turic, JT3 Photography – jt3photography.com

About the Author

John Simone has authored books for more than twenty five years. He has worked as an executive secretary, a computer programmer, and a technical writer and editor. He enjoys traveling and has been almost completely around the world. He underwent a Roux-en-Y gastric bypass in June 2007 and has maintained his goal weight for three years.

Other books by John Simone include:

Pcychic Awareness: Everything You Need to Know to Develop Your Psychic Abilities. ISBN-10: 1-886289-03-4. ISBN+13: 978-1-886289-03-1 Publication Date: 1995 176 pages .

The LCIS & DCIS Breast Cancer Fact Book. ISBN-10:: 1-886289-19-0. ISBN-13: 978-1-886289-19-2. Publication Date: March, 2002. 218 pages.

Astrology for Beginners. ISBN-10: 1-886289-13-1. ISBN+13 978-1-886289-13-0. Publication Date: 1995. 40 pages. Comb Bound.

The Intuitive Tarot Workbook. Workbook, comb bound. Available from Three Pyramids Publishing: http://www.three-pyramids.com/books.

Visit Our Website

Visit our website at http://www.three-pyramids.com for more information about bariatric surgery, links to other resources, and John's lectures and personal appearances.

Lectures and Personal Appearances

John Simone is available for lectures in your area. His talks are inspirational and motivational. John has led workshops on various topics in the USA and England.

Warning and Disclaimer

Special Sales

For information about bulk purchases or corporate premiums, please contact the Special Sales department at Three Pyramids Publishing, P.O.Box 432, Pine Plains, NY 12567-0432 USA.

Dedication

While having bariatric surgery was one of the best things I've ever done for myself, and one decision that I would never have done differently; the enormous lifestyle changes that it brought into my life were, for the most part, difficult and completely unexpected. I want to acknowledge those who helped me along the path.

To **Terry Smith**: you were beautiful when we met and you are beautiful now. Weight does not define beauty. Now you've had your surgery and have been at your goal weight for several years. Thank you for sharing your bariatric journey with me; it gave me the courage to have the surgery and make the necessary changes that kept me alive.

To **Rich Vasconi**: Lifelong friends are hard to find and harder to keep. It was so helpful to have someone with whom I could discuss the bariatric surgery. After my gastric hemorrhage, you made sure I had what I needed when I could not do for myself. You did all of the daily tasks that I could not handle with grace and generosity. Without your help, I could not have stayed in my home for the year that followed. Friends don't sign up to become caretakers, yet you did it without complaining or begrudging me the time lost from your own responsibilities.

To **Diane Simone Black** and **George Lefcheck**: thank you for taking me in after I became ill, and for slaving for years to give me a wonderful place to live. Words cannot express my gratitude.

To my **friends and family**, who always loved me, fat or thin!

Finally, to **bariatric patient**s everywhere – everyone's weight loss surgery journey is different, yet we all hope for the same thing: a healthier, longer, more active life. If you've tried to lose weight and keep it off before, you know how discouraging the process can be. Your surgery will give you the tool you lacked to get the excess pounds off and to change your life. I wish you much success!

Contents

Overview *1*

Your Life Will Change 3

Who Should Have Bariatric Surgery? 4

What is Body Mass Index (BMI)? 4

A Very Brief History of Weight Loss Surgery 5

Types of Bariatric Surgery 7

    Staged Procedures. 8

    Adjustable Gastric Band 9

        Advantages of Gastric Band Surgery. 11

        Disadvantages of Gastric Band Surgery 12

    Vertical Banded Gastroplasty 12

        Advantages of Vertical Banded Gastroplasty 13

        Disadvantages of Vertical Banded Gastroplasty. 13

    Vertical Sleeve Gastrectomy 15

        Advantages of Vertical Sleeve Gastrectomy 16

        Disadvantages of Vertical Sleeve Gastrectomy 16

    Gastric Bypass (Roux-en-Y). 17

        Advantages of Roux-en-Y Surgery 18

        Disadvantages of Roux-en-Y Surgery 19

    Biliopancreatic Diversion with Duodenal Switch 20

        Advantages of Biliopancreatic Diversion with Duodenal Switch Surgery. . 22

        Disadvantages of Biliopancreatic Diversion with Duodenal Switch Surgery 23

    Intragastric Balloon 23

        Advantages of Intragastric Balloon Surgery 24

        Disadvantages of Intragastric Balloon Surgery 24

Vagotomy 25

Implantable Gastric Stimulation 25

Jejunoileal Bypass 26

Reality Check 27

Bariatric Surgery is Not a Quick Fix. 28

Bariatric Surgery is Not Reversible 28

Expected Weight Loss Estimates 29

Myths *About Weight Loss Surgery*   *31*

What Not To Expect from Weight Loss Surgery 31

Being *Obese Hurts*   *33*

What Can You Do? 35

Improving *Co-morbid Conditions*   *37*

Eating *Disorders*   *39*

Bariatric Surgery and Binge Eating Disorders 39

Binge Eating 40

Night Eating Syndrome 40

Starvation Syndrome or Post-Surgical Eating Avoidance Disorder (PSEAD) . . . 41

Diet *and Lifestyle*   *43*

A Doctor Discusses Food and Diet 43

Diet and Lifestyle Changes 44

Lifestyle Changes After Bariatric Surgery 46

The Secret of Successful Weight Loss 49

Achieving and Maintaining the Ideal Weight 49

Determining a Baseline 50

Early Weight Loss 51

Overcoming a Weight Plateau 52

Weight Gain 53

    Minimizing Weight Gain After Bariatric Surgery. 54

    Reversing Weight Gain With Additional Surgery. 56

Insufficient Weight Loss 56

Developing New Diet and Eating Habits 57

Resources for Preparing Bariatric Meals 60

What Are Healthy Foods? 61

What About Portion Sizes? 62

What Not To Eat. 63

Signs of Problems With Bariatric Eating 64

Emotional Eating and Bariatric Surgery 65

Keep a Food Journal 66

Eating Away From Home After Bariatric Surgery 66

Exercise   *69*

    Start Slowly. 70

    Make an Activity Plan 71

    Join a Fitness Center 71

    Use a Personal Trainer 72

    Work Out With a Friend 73

    Exercise and Support Groups 73

Support *Groups*   *75*

Choosing a Support Group 77

Other Support Resources For Your New Lifestyle 79

Relationships *and Bariatric Surgery*   *81*

Coping With Relationship Changes .82

Romantic Relationships and Bariatric Surgery 84

Sex and the Bariatric Patient 85

Weight Loss Surgery and Body Image 86

Weight Loss Surgery and Fertility 86

Plastic *Surgery*   89

When To Have Plastic Surgery 92

Choosing a Plastic Surgeon. 94

Preventing Excess Skin. 95

Preventing Skin Surgery 95

Removing Excess Skin 96

Health Insurance and Excess Skin 99

Medicare 100

Medicaid and State-level Health Insurance 100

Body Contouring Surgical Procedures 100

Abdominoplasty 101

Arm Lift (Brachioplasty) 101

Augmentation Surgery. 102

Bicep and Tricep Augmentation. 102

Buttocks Lift and Buttocks Enhancement 103

Calf Implants 104

Pectoral Implants 104

Back Lift 105

Bra Line Back Lift 105

Breast Lift and Breast Implants 106

Face Lift 107

Liposuction 108

Lower Body Lift 108

Male Breast Reduction (Gynecomastia) 110

Neck Lift (Platysmaplasty) 112

Panniculectomy. 113

Thigh Lift 114

Potential Risks and Side Effects 115

What About Scars and Pain? 117

Potential *Problems After Weight Loss Surgery*   119

Complications Related To Co-morbid Conditions 119

Weight Loss Surgery and Food Addictions 120

Short Term Problems Following Surgery 121

Bleeding 121

Wound Infections 122

Blood Clots (Pulmonary Embolism) 122

Dysphagia (Difficulty in Swallowing) 123

Anastomotic Leaks 124

Staple Failure 124

Temporary Hair Loss 125

Thrush (Yeast Infection) 127

Problems That Develop Over Time 127

Dyspepsia (Indigestion) 128

Ulcers 128

Constipation 128

Hernia 129

Gallstones 129

Excess Skin 130

Feeling Cold 131

Gurgling Noises in the Abdomen 131

Dumping Syndrome 131

Bowel Obstruction 133

Diarrhea and Loose Stools (Steatorrhea) 134

Gas and Bloating 135

Flatulence 137

Lactose Intolerance 138

Stomal Stenosis 139

Food Blockage 139

Hyperparathyroidism 140

Protein Malnutrition 140

Calorie Malabsorption 142

Anemia 143

Achlorhydia 143

Osteoporosis 144

Alcohol Metabolism 144

Issues with Roux-en-Y or Biliopancreatic Diversion with Duodenal Switch . . 144

    Anastomotic Stricture 145

    Anastomotic Ulcers 145

Issues with Gastric Bands 146

    Gastric Band Erosion 146

    Gastric Band Slippage 146

    Malpositioning of the Gastric Band 147

    Problems with the Gastric Band Port 147

Vitamin *and Mineral Deficiencies*   *149*

Vitamin and Mineral Deficiencies 151

Vitamin A 152

Vitamin B1 (Thiamin) 153

Vitamin B7 (Biotin) 154

Vitamin B9 (Folate) 154

Vitamin B12 155

Vitamin D 156

Vitamin E 156

Vitamin H. 157

Mineral Deficiencies. 157

Calcium 157

Iron 157

Selecting Supplements 158

Pregnancy *After Bariatric Surgery*   *161*

Pregnancy and Complications of Obesity 162

Pregnancy Risks by Bariatric Surgery Type 163

Pregnancy and Bariatric Surgery 164

My *Weight Loss Story*   *167*

Hints, Tips and Personal Observations 175

Additional *Resources*   *177*

Organizations and Websites 178

Diet and Eating 178

Plastic Surgery 179

Bariatric Lifestyle 179

Finding footnote web references quoted in this book (PMIDs) 179

Index   *181*

1

Overview

A recent study from Blue Cross/Blue Shield found that more than one third (34%) of the non-institutionalized adult American population is obese — that's approximately 40 million people. Of this population, about 4 million are severely obese and 1.5 million are morbidly obese. Obesity contributes to about 300,000 deaths in this country each year. Health care costs associated with obesity amount to more than 100 billion dollars each year.

In the last decade, surgical procedures used to battle obesity have been researched, developed and refined.

More than 200,000 people had weight loss surgery in 2008, and hundreds of thousands more are considering it. Only about 1% of people who are candidates for weight loss surgery actually have the procedure each year.

Bariatric surgery, which is also called *weight loss surgery* (WLS), consists of several types of procedures performed on people who are dangerously obese in order to help them lose weight. This type of surgery can be *restrictive*, which prevents the intake of too large a quantity of food, or *malabsorptive*, which prevents the body from absorbing calories and other nutrients from the food that is ingested. Some bariatric procedures are both restrictive and malabsorptive.

Long term studies show that weight loss surgery offers significant long-term weight loss and medical improvement that can include recovery from diabetes, improvement in cardiovascular risk factors, and a reduction in mortality rate of 2.5% to 40%.[1]

Weight loss surgery is not a cure for obesity. The surgery enables dieting and exercising to finally work by controlling your appetite and making you feel full and satisfied with smaller amounts of food.

Every person who is considering weight loss surgery must understand that success is achieved not simply due to a surgical procedure; it requires a multidisciplinary team who can manage co–morbidities, nutrition, physical activity and exercise, behavior and psychological needs. The bariatric surgery itself is only a tool that helps to alter lifestyle and eating habits to achieve permanent weight loss.

Bariatric surgery requires a lifelong commitment to diet and nutritional issues. Every bariatric patient has to make several lifestyle changes — some of them quite significant — to ensure weight loss success. Some lifestyle changes actually begin before surgery, like quitting smoking, not drinking alcohol, losing 5 to 10% of excess body weight, and changing the way in which you eat (slow down, chew more, eat less).

Before your surgery, your bariatric surgeon required you to have a battery of tests that were done to uncover any pre-existing medical problems that might interfere with successful weight loss, or which necessitate procedural changes during surgery to ensure your safety. Others were psychological or behavior-related tests that are intended to help determine whether you are able to make the enormous lifestyle changes that bariatric surgery requires. Make no mistake: life after bariatric surgery changes drastically from what it was before surgery.

Bariatric teams attempt to cull people who think the surgery is a magic pill for weight loss: do this, and you'll be thin — no work required on your part. That path is a road to disaster when the patient discovers that eating all the cake you want after surgery is not an option. People who refuse to make lifestyle changes end up regaining most, if not all, of the weight they lost after bariatric surgery. Not only are they still overweight, they now have nutritional deficiencies and other issues that complicate life.

Even though every bariatric surgeon takes great pains to make you aware of what life will be like after surgery, this surgery is a shock to your

---

1   Malcolm K Robinson. Editorial, "Surgical Treatment of Obesity – Weighing the Facts." New England Journal of Medicine, July 30, 2009. 361:520. http://content.nejm.org/cgi/content/full/361/5/520.

system, both physically and emotionally. Life used to be centered on eating; now you eat only enough to survive. If you compare post-surgical portion sizes to what you ate before surgery, the portions will seem ridiculously tiny. Can anyone survive on such small amounts? Of course they can, and they do in many third world countries. Your friends and family, who are used to gorging at all-you-can-eat buffets in American restaurants, will tell you that you are not eating enough.

On a positive note, you will discover that you have incredible willpower — the same willpower you were convinced you lacked in the yo-yo diet days before your surgery. This is not a lifestyle change that wimps can handle. You will prove yourself to be strong and effective. You'll regain some of the self-respect you lost after years of being obese. Some friendships and other relationships will change. You must possess the inner strength to see the nay-sayers to the door while gathering your supporters closer. Some of your dearest friends will turn out to be not quite as supportive as you thought they would be; others will suddenly see you in a new light and treat you better than they did before. You might face jealousy or sexuality issues that will have to be resolved. You might suddenly discover that you do have a backbone and are no longer willing to take even the mildest forms of abuse, at home or at work.

People in your bariatric support group will also grow and begin to blossom before your eyes. The quiet older woman in our group who attended every meeting but knitted quietly in the corner and never spoke up is gone, and in her place is a happy, vibrant middle-aged woman with some very interesting tales to tell about her life. Your own insecurities will fade away.

You'll no longer have to worry about the ominous creak of a spindly wooden chair as you gingerly sit on it. There will actually be room for three people on your sofa. You can go for a boat ride without needing everyone else to sit on the opposite side to "balance you out."

These are the kinds of things that will make your weight loss successful over the long term.

Your Life Will Change

Make no mistake: everything about your life changes drastically after bariatric surgery, or is impacted in some way. Most bariatric patients agree that having weight loss surgery causes as much upheaval as getting married or having a baby — and that's before the weight loss begins. Many of these changes are completely unexpected, which makes them seem more important than they really are. You can expect to eat differently, see changes in your relationships, and your personality will change.

This book was written to help you cope with some of these issues.

Who Should Have Bariatric Surgery?

The National Institutes of Health recommends bariatric surgery for obese people with a body mass index (BMI) of at least 40, and for people who have a body mass index of 35 or more and serious coexisting medical conditions, such as diabetes.[2]

The American College of Physicians issued a medical guideline that concluded that surgery should be considered as a treatment option for patients with a BMI of 40 kg/m or greater who instituted but failed an adequate exercise and diet program (with or without adjunctive drug therapy) and who have obesity-related co-morbid conditions, such as hypertension, impaired glucose intolerance, diabetes mellitis, hyperlipidemia, and obstructive sleep apnea. A doctor-patient discussion of surgical options should include the long-term side effects, such as possible need for reoperation, gallbladder disease, and malabsorption. Patients should be referred to high-volume centers with surgeons experienced in bariatric surgery.[3, 4]

What is Body Mass Index (BMI)?

In the past, the term *morbid obesity* was applied to anyone who weighed more than 100 pounds more than the ideal body weight. Ideal body weight was determined by an actuarial table developed by the insurance industry that listed the weight at which one was estimated to live the longest. The tables were derived by averaging weight ranges for individuals of specific

---

2   Ibid.

3   V Snow, P Barry, N Fitterman, A Qaseem, K Weiss. "Pharmacologic and surgical management of obesity in primary care: a clinical practice guideline from the American College of Physicians." Ann. Intern. 2005. Med. 142 (7): 525–31. http://www.ncbi.nlm.nih.gov/pubmed/15809464

4   MA Maggard, LR Shugarman, M Suttorp, et al. "Meta-analysis: surgical treatment of obesity." Ann. Intern. 2005. Med. 142 (7): 547–59. http://www.ncbi.nlm.nih.gov/pubmed/15809466

height according to the number of years of life. This system did not predict accurately for shorter people.

In the 1990s, the National Institutes of Health convened a panel that investigated death rates using much more criteria than the insurance industry had used. The body mass index (BMI) was developed. The BMI is defined as the body weight (in kilograms) divided by the square of the height (in meters). The result is a number, usually between 20 and 70, in units of kilograms per square meter.

The panel recommended bariatric surgical treatment for individuals whose BMI was 40 or greater, and also for individuals with a BMI of 35 or greater with related co-morbid conditions like sleep apnea, diabetes, high cholesterol or high blood pressure. A person who has a BMI of 30 or greater is considered obese; people with BMI in the 30 to 35 range often can have gastric band surgery, which is effective for people with a BMI in that range. People in this group can achieve greater weight loss success than those who use only diet and exercise. Generally, bariatric surgeons will operate on people with a BMI over 40, since those people achieve the most benefits from bariatric surgery.

A *co-morbid condition* is a secondary illness or disease that affects a primary disease. Co-morbidities affect how the primary illness can be treated. In bariatric surgery, most patients have co-morbidities that must be considered before, during, and after the bariatric surgery.

While patients with co-morbidities can benefit from bariatric surgery, their additional conditions increase the risks associated with any surgery.

How to Determine Your BMI

Multiply your weight in pounds by 703. Divide the result by your height in inches. Divide that result by your height in inches again. The number that results is your BMI.

If your BMI is between 18.5 and 24.9, your weight is considered *normal*. A BMI of 25 to 29.9 is *overweight*. A BMI of 30 or more is considered *obese*.

A Very Brief History of Weight Loss Surgery

The original form of bariatric surgery was the jejunoileal bypass, originally performed in the 1950s at the University of Minnesota. The surgery created malabsorption while leaving the stomach intact. While most patients lost weight, most of them also developed serious complications related to malabsorption, including diarrhea, night blindness, osteoporosis, protein and calorie deficiencies, and kidney stones. Many patients also developed a toxic accumulation of bacteria in the bypassed section of the intestine, which subsequently caused liver failure, severe arthritis, skin problems, and flu-like symptoms. Because of the significant number of serious side effects, many jejunoileal patients required revisional surgery to reverse the procedure.

Jejunoileal bypass surgery is no longer performed in the USA. However, the history of patients who had the surgery informed current bariatric surgery. Surgeons today better understand the issues of malabsorption and what long-term effects to expect after weight loss surgery, which helps to reduce these problems after surgery today.

Gastric bypass surgery was developed in the 1960s after surgeons noticed beneficial weight loss in patients with stomach cancers who had part of their stomach removed. The surgery was originally done as a loop bypass, leaving most of the stomach intact. Problems with bile reflux resulted in development of the Roux-en-Y procedure, in which a limb of the intestine is connected to a very small stomach pouch and prevents bile from entering the stomach.

Gastroplasty was developed in the early 1970s as an alternative to jejunoileal bypass and Roux-en-Y surgery. The original surgery was made possible with the introduction of mechanical medical staplers. Nicknamed "stomach stapling," the procedure was completely restrictive. A horizontal line of surgical staples separated the stomach, creating a smaller upper pouch with a small unstapled opening that allowed food to move into the lower section and then through the natural digestive tract. The procedure was further developed as a vertical gastroplasty, in which a vertical small stomach pouch is created in the lesser curvature of the stomach and a Silastic™ ring is inserted at the outlet of the pouch. While the procedure results in fewer problems with malnutrition, weight regain has been a serious problem, and the procedure is rarely done now.

Biliopancreatic diversion surgeries were developed to take advantage of the malabsorption resulting from jejunoileal bypass, but offered a more controlled method for malabsorption. It reduced or eliminated much of the effect of toxic bacteria overgrowth associated with jejunoileal procedures. The biliopancreatic diversion with duodenal switch (BPDS) was developed to reduce the severity of protein and calorie malnutrition, increase the amount of gastric restriction, and minimize dumping syndrome. While biliopancreatic diversion with duodenal switch surgery offers the best long-term weight loss results, it also has the highest rate of nutritional complications of all weight loss surgeries. While many people consider the biliopancreatic diversion with duodenal switch a better alternative than the Roux-en-Y because of the lack of dumping syndrome, it also has some associated side effects, notably a low tolerance for fats that can result in diarrhea and excessive foul-smelling flatulence.

In 1994, surgeons began to use laparoscopic Roux-en-Y surgery, in which five or six small incisions are made in the abdomen. The abdominal cavity is inflated with carbon dioxide gas to make the internal organs more accessible. Surgical procedures are done using small instruments inserted into the incisions, with a viewing port containing a small camera in one of the openings used to guide the surgeon. Laparoscopic bariatric surgery offers fewer complications and a quicker recovery than open surgery, but not every patient is a good candidate for laparoscopic surgery, especially those with so much abdominal fat that the instruments cannot penetrate enough to work correctly, or with patients who have had significant previous abdominal surgery and subsequent internal scarring. In those cases, an open surgery must be used.

Adjustable gastric band surgery was developed to eliminate the need to resect the intestine or to cut into the stomach. It leaves the anatomy intact and works by restricting the quantity of food that can fit into a smaller stomach pouch. Since it is only a restrictive surgery, there are few side effects associated with malabsorptive procedures for this type of surgery, other than a possibility for calorie deficiency and productive burping if too much food is eaten too quickly.

Types of Bariatric Surgery

There are two forms of bariatric surgery: restrictive and malabsorptive.

Restrictive bariatric surgery reduces the size of the stomach. The smaller stomach pouch cannot hold large quantities of food, which prevents overeating. The uppermost portion of the stomach is believed to be the part that notifies the brain when we feel full after eating; restrictive surgery creates a much smaller food pouch that fills quickly and sends the appropriate signal to the brain.

Malabsorptive bariatric surgery curtails absorption of nutrients. While this method restricts the number of calories that can be absorbed from a meal, it also reduces the necessary vitamins, minerals and essential fatty acids that can be absorbed in the intestine.

Most of the modern bariatric procedures used today include both a restrictive and a malabsorptive method. Some surgeons use a mixed procedure of restrictive and malabsorptive techniques, based on the needs of the individual who is undergoing the surgery.

Restrictive procedures include:

✓ Vertical Banded Gastroplasty (VBG)

✓ Adjustable Gastric Band (also known as Lap Band)

✓ Sleeve Gastrectomy

✓ Intragastric balloon

Malabsorptive procedures include:

✓ Biliopancreatic Diversion

✓ Jejunoileal Bypass

Procedures which use both restrictive and malabsorptive methods include:

✓ Gastric Bypass (Roux-en-Y)

✓ Biliopancreatic Diversion with Duodenal Switch (also known as Sleeve Gastrectomy with Duodenal Switch)

In general, malabsorptive procedures result in greater weight loss than restrictive procedures.

All of these procedures result in short term weight loss. Some, such as jejunoileal bypass, have not withstood the test of time and other procedures have replaced them.

The three procedures commonly used today include Roux-en-Y, biliopancreatic diversion with duodenal switch, and gastric band. It is likely that you will have one of these three surgeries.

Staged Procedures

High-risk patients with severe obesity or significant medical co-morbid conditions can benefit from *staged bariatric procedures*. An initial surgery uses a less invasive procedure to help the patient begin losing weight. When enough weight is lost, or co-morbid conditions are brought under control, a second procedure is done that is more complex or definitive. The less invasive initial procedures include sleeve gastrectomy, gastric balloon and gastric band surgery, followed by the more complex Roux-en-Y or biliopancreatic diversion with duodenal switch.

Patients who qualify for weight loss surgery through a health insurance plan can usually have staged procedures approved if there is a medical need. The second surgery is done about a year after the first, on average; some surgeons will operate again within six months, but complete healing from the first surgery is usually a requirement before a second surgery can be performed.

Adjustable Gastric Band

This restrictive procedure uses an adjustable silicone band to reduce the size of the stomach. The band is placed around the top portion of the stomach to create a much smaller pouch. The remaining portion of the stomach is left as it is. This surgery is most commonly performed laparoscopically, and is commonly referred to as a "lap band" procedure for this reason.

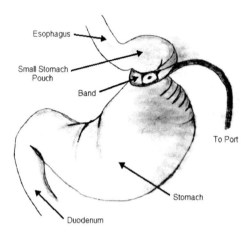

Esophagus

Small Stomach
Pouch

Band

To Port

Stomach

Duodenum

Adjustable Gastric Band

Unlike other bariatric surgeries, the stomach is not segmented or removed. The band can be removed, after which the stomach usually returns to its original state, making this type of bariatric surgery the only one that is reversible in a practical sense. However, it should not be considered as a reversible measure.

One major benefit is that it is an adjustable procedure. Your surgeon can tighten the gastric band to restrict food intake, or loosen it to allow more food. This benefit results in fewer nutritional issues than other forms of bariatric surgery. Another benefit is that only the surgeon can adjust the band, which improves the post-surgical rate of maintaining follow-up appointments and monitoring.

Because the surgery is relatively simple, it also has the fewest complication rates. It is almost always performed laparoscopically, which provides shorter recovery times. Gastric band surgery can be performed with a single incision instead of the usual four or five incisions needed for placement and visualization of the surgical site.

The tightness of the band can be changed by the addition or removal of saline solution into the band through a port installed just below the skin. The port is often placed in the navel area. The filling or draining technique is done by injection of sterile saline solution at the bariatric surgeon's office and is used to control how much food can be ingested. This process controls how quickly you lose weight.

Overeating often causes vomiting, since the stomach can only accept a limited amount of food at one time. As with other bariatric surgeries, do not drink fluids with meals. Drinking while eating food increases the possibility for nausea, discomfort and vomiting, and helps the food to move out of the stomach pouch too quickly.

This procedure is often performed on people within the lower BMI range. It has also been used on people with a very high BMI coupled with significant co-morbidities in order to get their weight down enough so that a more comprehensive bariatric procedure can be performed as their health improves. While health insurance companies don't like to pay for the same type of surgery twice, it is sometimes medically necessary and can be justified on that basis.

One common problem after gastric banding is called *productive burping*, the occasional regurgitation of food or saliva. It is often a symptom of eating too quickly or not chewing food enough.

Life after gastric band surgery is relatively uncomplicated for most patients. The small stomach pouch severely restricts the amount of food that can be eaten at one time.

If you eat too much or too quickly, you can stretch the stomach pouch slightly. This enables you to eat progressively larger meals. If this happens, your bariatric surgeon can adjust the amount of saline filling the band to make it more restrictive. The band can also be shifted surgically to a different position to create a smaller stomach pouch, although this is not usually necessary for most people. As with any of the weight loss surgeries, eating less is the basis for successful weight loss and in maintaining your ideal weight.

Advantages of Gastric Band Surgery

Gastric band surgery has several advantages over other types of bariatric surgery:

✓ It is adjustable

✓ It is reversible (with some restrictions)

✓ The surgery is less invasive

✓ Gastric band surgery can be done on an outpatient basis with no hospital stay

✓ It results in fewer nutritional deficiencies, since it does not interfere with absorption

✓ There is no risk of dumping syndrome

✓ It improves co-morbid health problems, such as type 2 diabetes, sleep apnea, high cholesterol, high blood pressure and asthma

✓ Weight loss is slow and steady

Some patients, however, have only moderate weight loss with gastric band surgery, or achieve almost no significant weight loss. A study by researchers associated with the University of California at San Francisco reported in the Archives of Surgery released in September 2008 found that for some individuals, the deck might be stacked against them. This group includes diabetics and those whose surgery resulted in the creation of a stomach pouch that was too large.

People with diabetes take insulin and other drugs that stimulate the production of fat and cholesterol. Other factors include their tendency toward a reactive increase in calorie intake to counteract episodes of hypoglycemia, a reduction of urinary glucose losses, and water retention that is a direct result of insulin use.

Additionally, bariatric surgeons size the stomach pouch subjectively. They size the new stomach pouch using anatomical landmarks instead of using a sizing balloon. The size of the new stomach pouch restricts the amount of food the patient can consume; larger pouches allow more food to be ingested. Efforts are under way to provide ways to size the stomach pouch more accurately.

Disadvantages of Gastric Band Surgery

Gastric band surgery also has some disadvantages:

✓ Total weight loss is usually less than with other procedures (although over time, weight loss rates compare favorably with other procedures)

✓ Weight is lost more slowly

✓ The size of the stomach pouch varies from patient to patient, affecting results

✓ Productive burping can be an issue

Vertical Banded Gastroplasty

Vertical banded gastroplasty, which used to be known as "stomach stapling," is a restrictive procedure used for weight control. It was developed in 1980 and was in vogue as the bariatric surgery of choice for ten to fifteen years. Both a band and staples are used to create a smaller stomach pouch. A one centimeter hole is left at the base of the pouch, through which the contents of the stomach pouch can pass into the rest of the stomach, then through the pyloric valve into the duodenum. Some surgeons use a polypropylene mesh band or a Silastic band around the opening to prevent enlargement or staple failure.

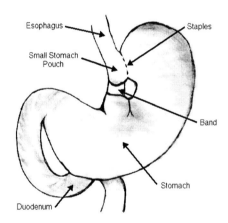

Vertical Banded Gastroplasty

The technique both restricts the quantity of food that can be consumed and slows its passage out of the stomach.

This form of bariatric surgery is slowly being replaced by gastric band procedures. Gastric band procedures do not require cutting into the stomach and do not use lines of staples, making it a safer alternative.

The American Medical Association has classified vertical banded gastroplasty as a "severely dangerous" surgical procedure because of the high rates of complications and infections.

Advantages of Vertical Banded Gastroplasty

Vertical banded gastroplasties have these advantages:

✓ fewer nutritional deficiencies since it is not malabsorptive

✓ a lower mortality rate

✓ patients do not develop dumping syndrome

Disadvantages of Vertical Banded Gastroplasty

Vertical banded gastroplasty has significant disadvantages:

✓ 1 patient in 100 dies from complications from this surgery within a year

✓ Reversal surgery is difficult and presents additional complications

✓ Patients must follow a strict diet to achieve success

✓ Regaining weight is common

✓ Many patients suffer from extreme heartburn

✓ High fiber foods and foods with a dense natural consistency are harder to digest than highly refined foods. This means that healthier foods are harder to digest than junk foods, which encourages weight regain after surgery.

✓ Bariatric surgery that is only restrictive in nature requires strict adherence to post-surgical diet and exercise plans.

✓ While vertical banded gastroplasty can be reversed, the revisional surgery is much more complicated than the original procedure. If the band is removed after a period of a few years, it is likely that significant scar tissue has developed at the band site. This area of scar tissue in the stomach often needs to be removed. When the line of staples is removed, the two parts of the stomach that were separated must be rejoined by stitching them together. Revisional surgery is usually considered only when there is a serious medical complication that warrants it.

✓ Eating food too quickly or not chewing food enough can more easily cause vomiting and discomfort than other procedures

✓ Patients do not develop dumping syndrome, so those who have a fondness for sweets can continue to eat them in excess

✓ Unlike gastric band procedures, the band is not adjustable.

After vertical banded gastroplasty, there is a risk that the stomach pouch could stretch and become larger, in some cases becoming as large as the entire stomach was originally. The food pouch doubles in size in the first two months after this surgery. The line of surgical staples can be strained to the point where they break open, which effectively enlarges the stomach to its original size. In addition, leakage of the stomach acids into the abdomen can seriously damage other organs. If the contents of the stomach move too quickly into the gastrointestinal tract, it can result in nausea, bloating, diarrhea or discomfort.

There is also a chance, as with other bariatric surgery, for hernia or developing gallstones.

Vertical Sleeve Gastrectomy

A sleeve gastrectomy is a restrictive weight loss surgery in which the stomach is reduced to about 15% of its original size. It is a variation of biliopancreatic diversion with duodenal switch. The larger curvature is isolated by a series of vertical staples, or is removed completely. The remaining section is a vertical sleeve or tube that connects the top of the stomach where the esophagus enters to the bottom of the stomach, where the intestines begin.

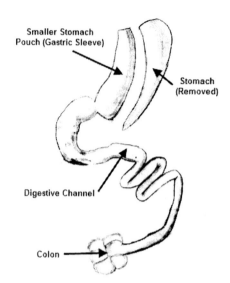

Smaller Stomach Pouch (Gastric Sleeve)

Stomach (Removed)

Digestive Channel

Colon

Vertical Sleeve Gastrectomy

As with other bariatric surgeries, the procedure is not reversible. It can be performed laparoscopically.

This type of bariatric surgery is useful for people with pre-existing anemia, Crohn's Disease, or other physical conditions that make them too high a risk for other (primarily malabsorptive) weight loss surgeries.

Sleeve gastrectomy is often performed as the first step in a two-part staged procedure for people whose BMI is 50 or higher, in which the risk of performing a gastric bypass or duodenal switch is too great. This form of surgery is an excellent first step that is used to bring their weight down into a less dangerous range, to make possible a secondary type of weight loss surgery (often Roux-en-Y or biliopancreatic diversion with duodenal switch) that can be done if not enough weight is lost. It is also used independently because of the lack of problems associated with nutrient malabsorption.

The pylorus at the base of the stomach remains intact after surgery. The pyloric valve is a ring of muscle at the end of the pylorus that allows food to pass at a controlled rate from the stomach into the duodenum. Because the pyloric function and duodenum are not bypassed in sleeve gastrectomies, the issues that affect malabsorptive procedures do not occur with this weight loss surgery.

Because it is a restrictive procedure, weight loss can be lost less rapidly than with other procedures. However, long–term success rates after this surgery are higher.

Advantages of Vertical Sleeve Gastrectomy

Vertical sleeve gastrectomy has several advantages:

✓ It can be used as an interim surgery for patients to begin losing weight but who are not good candidates medically for other weight loss surgeries

✓ The pyloric valve remains intact after surgery, resulting in a more normal flow of food from the stomach into the duodenum

✓ The duodenum is left intact; nutrients and calories are absorbed much as they were before surgery

✓ Patients do not develop dumping syndrome

✓ Patients do not develop nutrition problems associated with malabsorptive procedures

✓ It has a high long–term success rate

✓ The surgery can be performed laparoscopically

Disadvantages of Vertical Sleeve Gastrectomy

Disadvantages of vertical sleeve gastrectomy include:

✓ Weight loss is less rapid than with other bariatric procedures

✓ The surgery is not reversible

Gastric Bypass (Roux-en-Y)

Gastric bypass procedures account for a large majority of bariatric surgeries performed in the USA today, with more than 200,000 procedures performed each year.

There are several forms of this surgery, differing mainly in how the connections are made between stomach and bowel and between bowel sections. The most common form is the Roux-en-Y gastric bypass.

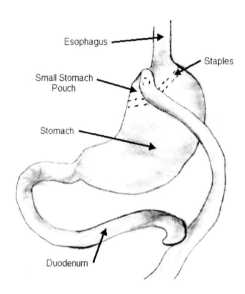

Esophagus

Staples

Small Stomach
Pouch

Stomach

Duodenum

Roux-en-Y Gastric Bypass

In the Roux-en-Y procedure, a very small thumb-sized pouch is created at the top of the stomach. The rest of the stomach is bypassed using staples or sutures. This provides a significant restriction in the amount of food that can be eaten. Then the gastrointestinal tract is reconstructed in a way that induces malabsorption. Variations of gastric bypass surgery involving different methods for reconnecting the gastrointestinal tract can be used to vary the amount and type of malabsorption.

Food is processed through the stomach pouch into the digestive limb of the small intestine. The shorter loop connected to the base of the old stomach, which is no longer used for delivery of partly digested food, receives bile from the liver. The two sections are rejoined further along the gastrointestinal tract, allowing food and bile to combine for digestion. Where this junction is made to the small intestine determines the amount of nutrients that are absorbed. If the junction is done higher in the gastrointestinal tract (about 18" below the stomach), the procedure is known as a proximal Roux-en-Y; if it is done lower along the tract (usually 40-60" from the lower end of the bowel), it is a distal Roux-en-Y.

Distal Roux-en-Y procedures deliver slightly better weight losses, but the process of dumping undigested food so far along into the gastrointestinal tract produces more irritants and malodorous gas.

Most Roux-en-Y surgeries are performed laparoscopically. It is not considered to be a reversible surgery since several anatomical changes are made. The length of the intestinal pathways can be changed, but cannot be restored to pre–surgical condition.

Advantages of Roux-en-Y Surgery

Roux-en-Y surgery has several benefits over other forms of weight loss surgeries:

✓ Ghrelin, the hormone that triggers feelings of hunger, is produced in the greater curvature of the stomach. This portion is sectioned off from the digestive tract. Roux-en-Y patients rarely feel hungry even after severely limiting the amount of food they ingest.

✓ About 90% of type 2 diabetics are cured (become euglycemic) almost immediately after the surgery, due to the metabolic changes caused by the intestinal rerouting.

✓ The combination of moderate restriction on the amount of food that can be ingested, along with the major malabsorption, causes the loss of 65 to 80% of excess body weight, and has a lowered risk of regaining the lost weight.

✓ Major reduction in co-morbidities after Roux-en-Y include 90% for type 2 diabetes, 70% for hyperlipidemia (high blood cholesterol), 90% or greater for sleep apnea, and 70% for hypertension (high blood pressure). Both diabetes and sleep apnea have been reported to be cured by Roux-en-Y surgery.

✓ Gastroesophageal reflux disease (GERD), a condition in which the contents of the stomach pass back into the esophagus, is relieved immediately after surgery in almost all patients.

✓ Venous thromboembolic diseases, such as swelling in the legs, are much improved.

✓ Low back pain and bone joint pain is alleviated in most patients.

✓ A recent study in mortality rates across a large population of post-bariatric patients revealed an 89% drop in mortality rates as opposed to patients with the same medical profiles who were not treated surgically.

✓ Roux-en-Y patients often develop dumping syndrome, which helps them avoid foods that are high in sugars (and the associated risk of weight regain from those foods).

Disadvantages of Roux-en-Y Surgery

There are also disadvantages associated with Roux-en-Y:

✓ Dumping syndrome is experienced by a large number of Roux-en-Y patients.

✓ The stomach pouch that is created during surgery can expand slightly over time, allowing greater food intake that reduces the effectiveness of the restrictive aspect of the surgery.

✓ Because Roux-en-Y surgery is malabsorptive, patients have to take vitamin and mineral supplements for the rest of their lives, in quantity or strength that is beyond what is required by the normal population. This is not optional and it will continue for the rest of their life.

✓ Extensive annual blood testing is needed to monitor for nutritional deficiencies.

✓ Gallstones caused by rapid weight loss are commonly seen after Roux-en-Y surgeries. Many bariatric surgeons routinely remove the gallbladder during the bariatric surgery as a preventive measure. If it was not removed before surgery, there is a good chance that it will have to be removed in the future. Medication might also be required to reduce the production of gallstones.

A Roux-en-Y procedure reduces stomach capacity by more than 90%. The stomach pouch is created from the upper area of the stomach, which is less prone to stretching to a larger size. This resistance to stretching, along with its small original size, help to prevent the stomach pouch from expanding over time. Note, however, that the small intestine can stretch slightly to hold more food as time passes.

Roux-en-Y patients have a sense of feeling full after eating only a very small amount of food after surgery. They learn quickly that continuing to eat is an invitation to feeling uncomfortable or vomiting. Taking smaller bites and eating slowly can help prevent this issue.

Some Roux-en-Y patients are told to eat only 3 small meals daily and to avoid all snacks between meals. Others are advised to eat 4 to 6 very small meals daily, spreading food intake out over the course of the day. With Roux-en-Y surgeries, weight usually is not regained because the stomach has stretched, since the capacity for food has not changed, but instead because of high-calorie snacking or excessive or constant eating (a behavior sometimes called *grazing*).

Dumping Syndrome is one complication not seen in other types of bariatric surgeries. It is a significant issue that must be factored into the decision to have this form of bariatric surgery. Dumping syndrome is characterized by a lowered tolerance to simple sugars, which cause considerable digestive upset, pain and diarrhea. Since many overweight people are seriously addicted to sugars, dumping syndrome is an effective, if unpleasant, side effect that helps them curb their affection for sweets. For more information on dumping syndrome, see "Dumping Syndrome" on page 131.

Biliopancreatic Diversion with Duodenal Switch

Biliopancreatic diversion surgeries were used in the late 1990s and into the 21st century. It has been replaced by a modified version, the biliopancreatic diversion with duodenal switch. The surgery was modified to help combat several issues related to malnourishment.

The biliopancreatic diversion with duodenal switch procedure, also called *Sleeve Gastrectomy* or *Gastric Reduction Duodenal Switch* surgery, is a weight loss surgery procedure that is both restrictive and malabsorptive.

The restrictive portion involves bypassing about 70% of the stomach. If the surgeon creates a vertical sleeve separated from the remaining stomach by staples or sutures, the surgery is a *sleeve gastrectomy with duodenal switch*. In a biliopancreatic diversion with duodenal switch, the excess portion of the stomach is completely removed. Both methods are equally effective. Individual surgeons determine whether the stomach is removed or simply bypassed, depending on the circumstances presented by each patient.

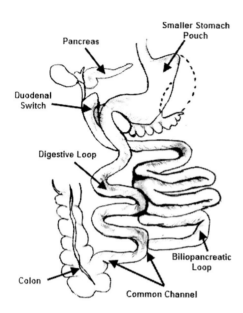

Biliopancreatic Diversion with Duodenal Switch

The malabsorptive portion reroutes a large part of the small intestine, creating two separate pathways and a common channel. The much longer pathway, the biliopancreatic loop, carries bile from the liver to the common channel. The smaller channel carries partly digested food from the smaller stomach pouch to the common channel. The bile from the biliopancreatic loop channel combines with the contents of the digestive channel in the short common channel before it moves into the large intestine. This method reduces the amount of time the body has to extract calories from food, while selectively limiting the absorption of fat. Only about 20% of the fat that is ingested is absorbed.

While this procedure can be performed laparoscopically, it is more frequently done as an open surgery in the USA. Surgeons using laparoscopic biliopancreatic diversion with duodenal switch procedures must be accomplished and very experienced at doing the procedure.

About 2% of biliopancreatic diversion with duodenal switch patients need to have their surgery revised each year because of severe malnutrition.

Biliopancreatic diversion with duodenal switch patients are able to enjoy a diet that most resembles a normal diet after surgery. They can have issues with too much fat in their diet, which can cause diarrhea and excessive foul-smelling flatulence.

Advantages of Biliopancreatic Diversion with Duodenal Switch Surgery

Biliopancreatic diversion with duodenal switch has several benefits over other forms of weight loss surgeries:

✓ The pyloric valve at the base of the stomach is maintained. This prevents the dumping syndrome common after Roux-en-Y procedures. Food is processed through the stomach in a more normal manner.

✓ Fewer problems with food intolerance develop than with other bariatric procedures.

✓ Ulcers are less common with this procedure.

✓ Biliopancreatic diversion with duodenal switch patients follow a more normal diet with fewer restrictions than patients using other weight loss surgery procedures.

✓ Ghrelin, the hormone that triggers feelings of hunger, is produced in the greater curvature of the stomach. This portion is sectioned off from the digestive tract. Biliopancreatic diversion with duodenal switch patients rarely feel hungry even after severely limiting the amount of food they ingest.

✓ About 98% of type 2 diabetics are cured (become euglycemic) almost immediately after the surgery, due to the metabolic changes caused by the intestinal switch. This effect is so widespread that surgeons in Europe are using the duodenal switch on patients of normal body size in an effort to cure diabetes.

✓ The combination of moderate restriction on the amount of food that can be ingested, along with the major malabsorption, causes a very high percentage of excess weight loss combined with a very low risk of regaining the lost weight.

✓ Major reduction in co-morbidities after biliopancreatic diversion with duodenal switch include 90-99% for type 2 diabetes, 70-99% for hyperlipidemia (high blood cholesterol), 92% for sleep apnea, and 70-83% for hypertension (high blood pressure).

✓ The effects of obstructive sleep apnea are significantly reduced. Sleep apnea is often reported to be cured after surgery.

Disadvantages of Biliopancreatic Diversion with Duodenal Switch Surgery

There are also disadvantages associated with biliopancreatic diversion with duodenal switch:

✓ The stomach pouch that is created during surgery can expand over time, allowing greater food intake, which reduces the effectiveness of the restrictive aspect of the surgery.

✓ Because biliopancreatic diversion with duodenal switch surgery is malabsorptive, you will have to take vitamin and mineral supplements in a quantity or strength that is beyond what is required by the normal population. This is not optional and it will continue for the rest of your life.

✓ Ulcers can develop, but are less common than with other forms of bariatric surgery (particularly Roux-en-Y).

✓ Extensive (and potentially expensive) annual blood testing is needed to monitor for nutritional deficiencies.

✓ Vitamin A deficiencies can cause night blindness.

✓ Gallstones caused by rapid weight loss are commonly seen after biliopancreatic diversion with duodenal switch surgeries. Many bariatric surgeons routinely remove the gallbladder during the bariatric surgery as a preventive measure. If it was not removed before surgery, there is a good chance that it will have to be removed in the future. Medication might also be required to reduce the production of gallstones.

Intragastric Balloon

Note: This type of bariatric surgery is not approved for use in the USA.

While this form of weight loss surgery is not used in the USA, it is used in many countries in Europe and South America. It is commonly used in Canada, Australia, Mexico and India.

The surgical procedure is done under sedation or general anesthesia in an outpatient facility. A deflated balloon is placed into the stomach endoscopically and then inflated with liquid or air to decrease the amount of space available inside the stomach for food. It is inflated using a catheter that is passed through the endoscope. The balloon is self-sealing when the catheter is removed and floats freely in the stomach. It is too large to be regurgitated or to pass into the intestine.

No incision is made through the skin. The entire process is done through an endoscope, which is inserted through the mouth and down the esophagus.

The balloon is usually removed after about six months and results in the loss of 5-9 BMI units.

Current guidelines indicate that patients with a lower BMI of 27 or more are candidates for intragastric balloon surgery.

Most patients regain between 25 and 40% of their lost weight within a year; this is often because their eating habits did not change after the procedure.

There is a slight chance that the balloon can be deflated while it is in position in the stomach, which can require surgical removal. Otherwise, it is removed using an endoscopic procedure. Placement and removal procedures can be done using very mild sedation, and it is considered a relatively low impact surgery.

Advantages of Intragastric Balloon Surgery

✓ No abdominal incisions are made; the surgery is performed via endoscope

✓ A temporary solution, it is removed after about six months

✓ It is completely reversible

✓ Can be done with mild or no sedation; general anesthesia is not required (but can be used)

✓ Patients with BMIs too low for other bariatric surgery can benefit

Disadvantages of Intragastric Balloon Surgery

✓ It is restrictive and a temporary solution; the restriction lasts only as long as the balloon is inflated and in place

✓ Lower overall weight loss due to the short period in which it is used

✓ The balloon can deflate spontaneously or from sharp food particles and would have to be removed

Vagotomy

The use of vagotomy as a form of bariatric surgery is currently being studied. It has been used in other parts of the world, but is not yet an accepted bariatric surgery in the USA. A vagotomy is a surgical procedure that involves the partial removal of the vagus nerve that services organs in the abdominal cavity.[5] While studies indicate that the amount of weight that can potentially be lost after a vagotomy is much less than with current bariatric procedures, advocates say it has a potential application in the future.

Early results from the studies show an average of 18% weight loss[6], significantly less than with other bariatric procedures. The procedure is neither restrictive nor malabsorptive; results are more difficult to achieve and are attainable only if a prescribed diet is strictly followed. Weight regain is a common problem.

The vagus nerve is rarely completely severed. Instead, a partial vagotomy is performed, which affects only the part of the vagus nerve that impacts the stomach. Additional sections of the vagus service the intestinal tract, which is negatively affected after complete vagotomy.[7]

One healthy side effect of vagotomy is that it reduces acid production in the stomach, which is a boon for people suffering from gastric ulcers and subsequent ulcer perforation. It also reduces gastroesophageal reflux. Patients lose the sensation of being hungry.

---

5   Lauren Neergaard. "Could Nerve-Snipping Spur Weight Loss?" USA Today. 7/2/2007. http://www.usatoday.com/news/health/2007-07-02-obesity-nerve-snip_N.htm

6   Kimberly Tere. "Vagotomy: Is cutting the vagus nerve the answer to weight loss?" Gastric Bypass Surgery News, May 12, 2008. http://www.usatoday.com/news/health/2007-07-02-obesity-nerve-snip_N.htm

7   PH Jordan, J Thornby "Twenty years after parietal cell vagotomy or selective vagotomy antrectomy for treatment of duodenal ulcer. Final report." Ann. Surg. September 2004. 220 (3): 283–293; discussion 293–296. http://www.ncbi.nlm.nih.gov/pubmed/8092897

Implantable Gastric Stimulation

Note: This procedure is not currently approved for use in the USA.

Implantable gastric stimulation involves surgically implanting a device similar to a heart pacemaker in the stomach, with the electrical leads stimulating the external surface of the stomach. The electrical stimulation modifies the activity of the enteric nervous system of the stomach, which stimulates the brain in feeling satiated or full. The procedure is neither restrictive nor malabsorptive. It is considered to be reversible.

Current studies conclude that it is less effective than other forms of bariatric surgery. It is not likely it will become an approved surgical methodology in the USA.

Jejunoileal Bypass

Note: This type of bariatric surgery is no longer performed in the USA.

Jejunoileal bypass surgery was performed from the mid-1950s until late in the 1970s. This open surgery resulted in the flow of food from the stomach bypassing the entire jejunum, connecting directly with the ileum, which is the last 12 to 18 inches of the small intestine.

The jejunum is the very long middle section of the small intestine. The ileum is the shorter part that connects the small intestine with the large intestine. The normal length of the small intestine is 20 feet. The jejunum, which had no upstream flow from the stomach, often developed dangerous bacterial infections (sepsis) that needed to be treated surgically.

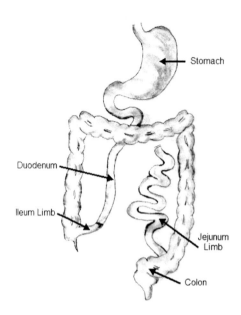

Jejunoileal Bypass

Almost all jejunoileal bypass surgeries were reversed as patients developed severe malnutrition and life-threatening septic infections.

Post surgical patients suffered from many malabsorptive issues, including malnutrition and liver failure. They also presented vitamin, mineral, protein, fat and essential acid deficiencies. The fatty acids that discharged into the intestine irritated the colon walls and caused secretion of excessive volumes of water and electrolytes (especially sodium and potassium), resulting in diarrhea. Most jejunoileal bypass patients had significant problems with constant or excessive diarrhea, often occurring five or more times each day. There were also issues with the rapid creation of gallstones.

Patients also reported a significant amount of pain.

On a positive note, the malabsorptive issues caused by jejunoileal bypass enabled the medical community to develop the newer forms of weight loss surgery. Bariatric surgeons now know what issues to expect as a result of a malabsorptive procedure and can ensure that measures are taken to mitigate their effects.

Reality Check

Americans have become an impatient people. Because of technological advances, much of what occurs today happens quickly, and we have come to expect equally fast results in everything we do.

Bariatric surgeons cringe when a prospective patient tells them how excited they are at the prospect of "losing all that extra weight so quickly and so effortlessly."

Weight loss is not an effortless process, whether bariatric surgery is used or not. After surgery, your lifestyle must change. Your eating habits must change, both in terms of quantity and types of food. You will not end up looking like you did twenty years ago.

Weight loss surgery is simply a tool that will make it less difficult to lose weight. It is not a solution in itself. It's not magic — it's work!

With other forms of addictions, you can continue to live and thrive without drugs, alcohol or cigarettes. Food is different; there is no way to escape having to eat every day. After your surgery, you must still focus on losing weight and maintaining your weight loss. Bariatric surgery simply creates physical changes that make it easier to change negative dietary habits into more healthy ones.

Will you lose all of your excess weight? Some patients are able to reach a normal weight, while others will remain slightly overweight but be less obese than before surgery. Success in reaching the goal weight is based on a realistic appraisal of your final goal weight, how compliant you are with diet and exercise, and how committed you are to making the weight loss process a success. Maintaining your goal weight requires commitment to lifestyle and diet changes, increased exercise, and better food choices over the long term. Success cannot be achieved if you revert to eating the way you did before surgery.

Bariatric Surgery is Not a Quick Fix

Bariatric surgery is not a quick fix for obesity. It is a permanent process used to resolve the issue of weight gain and should be performed when more traditional weight loss methods, such as increased exercise and reduction of food intake, are ineffective.

If you have co-morbid conditions, many are likely to improve after bariatric surgery, and some, like type 2 diabetes or sleep apnea, might resolve completely. However, over the years, those conditions have caused other issues. For example, type 2 diabetes often promotes kidney damage or failure. Damaged organs cannot regenerate to like-new condition. While the co-morbid condition appears to be resolved, there are still consequences as time progresses for having had the co-morbidity at all. Bariatric surgery does not fix that problem.

Bariatric Surgery is Not Reversible

While some forms of bariatric surgery can be revised, most result in anatomical changes that cannot be reversed. The adjustable gastric band can be removed and the entire stomach remains viable, but in practical terms, the stomach will probably not be in the same condition as one that was not banded. Overeating can stress the smaller stomach pouch above the band, causing scar tissue to form that remains after band removal. The scar tissue causes restriction as if the band were still in place, although to a lesser degree, and removing the scar tissue is a relatively difficult surgical procedure.

The other forms of bariatric surgery are not considered reversible. While surgical revision is possible, the stomach and intestines cannot be returned to the same condition as before surgery. Bariatric surgery results in permanent changes.

Expected Weight Loss Estimates

Weight Loss Surgery	Pounds Lost 3 Years After Surgery
Biliopancreatic Diversion with Duodenal Switch	117
Roux-en-Y	90
Gastric Band	77
Sleeve Gastrectomy	79
Notes: • More recent studies have shown that the medium (3-8 years) and long-term (more than 10 years) weight loss results for Roux-en-Y and Gastric Band surgeries become very similar. • Data beyond five years for Sleeve Gastrectomy is not yet available (as of 2009)	

2

Myths About Weight Loss Surgery

It is easy to get caught up in the excitement of having bariatric surgery, and people contemplating it are more than a little optimistic about the end results. Even though most bariatric surgeons are thorough about discussing the long-term effects of the surgery, patients focus on the information about the positive outcome and ignore much of the rest of the information that was given to them.

Maintaining your optimism is a good thing. However, you have to realize that much of what you anticipate to be the end result of the surgery might not work out according to plan. Weight loss surgery is not a magical procedure. Advertising provided by bariatric surgeons point out that "pounds will melt away" after the surgery, but it is rarely noted that it still requires significant effort of your part to achieve and maintain success.

What Not To Expect from Weight Loss Surgery

Here are some myths about weight loss surgery to keep in mind:

Weight loss is an easy solution to my weight problem. Bariatric surgery is not a magic pill. It's a tool that enables you to lose weight after surgery by restricting your caloric intake, using malabsorption, restriction, or a combination of both. This makes it easier to lose weight, but success is determined by your ability to make dietary and lifestyle changes that support the weight loss.

I'll look like I did when I graduated high school / got married / before I had my first baby. You might end up weighing the same as you did then, but Mother Nature has some nasty tricks up her sleeve. As time passes, gravity takes its toll, your skin ages, and you end up looking quite different even at the same weight.

I'll lose 100% of my excess weight. You almost certainly will not shed 100% of your excess weight. You're not going to reach your ideal weight as a result of surgery. You might achieve your ideal weight if you maintain your dietary and exercise plans for the rest of your life

Life will be easy. Let's face it: life before bariatric surgery was not easy. Just being thin doesn't make life easy. If anything, you'll have more stamina and getting through the day will be a simpler task. However, the same life issues and problems you had before surgery exist after surgery.

Bariatric surgery will make me thin. Bariatric surgery can help patients lose upwards of 50% of their excess body fat. However, most bariatric patients lose only about 75 to 80% of their total excess body weight. For example, patients who are 150 pounds overweight often can still be about 50 pounds overweight at the end of the process. It is essential that you understand the limitations of bariatric surgery. This is why, before your surgery, you are required to consult with a psychologist or other mental health professional.

Bariatric surgery is a once in a lifetime event. Weight-loss surgery is a lifetime relationship between surgeon and patient. Much of your weight loss success is a result of what happens after the surgery. After any weight loss surgical procedure, you'll meet annually with your bariatric team for blood tests and other evaluations, and the effort you take in following up after surgery is directly related to your long–term success.

I can eat whatever I want. Your anatomy is different after weight loss surgery. There are going to be some foods — and it can be quite a long list — that you cannot tolerate after surgery. You can continue to eat them if you don't mind feeling terrible afterward. Almost all bariatric patients, however, quickly determine that no single food is that important to them. No human can gorge on high calorie foods and not gain weight.

3

Being Obese Hurts

If you contemplated bariatric surgery, you already know that being obese is harmful.

The effects of obesity are far ranging. A study reported by the American Council of Science and Health listed a few.[1]

Obesity:

✓ is unattractive

✓ shortens your life span by six or seven years, or more if you have several co-morbid conditions

✓ dramatically increases the chances of developing hypertension (high blood pressure), a leading cause of coronary disease and stroke

✓ impairs breathing due to the excess fat tissue around the ribs and abdomen

✓ increases your risk of developing asthma

✓ causes sleep apnea, a condition in which people stop breathing for several seconds while asleep

✓ increases your risk for developing uterine, colon, esophageal and male and female breast cancer

---

1   Elizabeth Whelan. "A Consumer Guide to Bariatric Surgery: The Lesser Known Effects of Obesity." April 4, 2009. https://www.acsh.org/healthissues/newsID.1795/healthissue_detail.asp

- ✓ is linked to an increase in the risk for prostate, ovarian, liver, thyroid and stomach cancers

- ✓ increases your risk for developing multiple myeloma and non-Hodgkin's lymphoma

- ✓ increases your risk for developing gallstones and kidney stones

- ✓ increases your risk of complications from anesthesia used during surgery, even for routine sedation dentistry

- ✓ increases your risk of post-surgical infection

- ✓ increases the risk for needing gall bladder surgery

- ✓ increases complications of pregnancy, including gestational diabetes and high blood pressure

- ✓ can cause delays in becoming pregnant

- ✓ can cause infertility in both males and females

- ✓ is associated with a lower viable sperm count in males

- ✓ can cause urinary incontinence and erectile dysfunction in males

- ✓ increases the risk of developing Parkinson's Disease in both men and women

- ✓ increases the risk of developing inflammatory skin diseases and psoriasis

- ✓ increases the risk of accidental injury, since obese people are more prone to falling and other accidents

Unfortunately, being obese subjects you to all of these risks.

What Can You Do?

There are several steps you can take now to begin reducing the negative effects of obesity.

✓ Determine your body mass index (BMI) and reduce that number. If your BMI is over 25, you are overweight. If it is 30 or higher, you are obese. If it is 40 or more, you are morbidly obese and your life span is affected.

✓ Understand and act upon the fact that the number of calories you consume each day and the amount of activity you do to burn those calories determines your weight loss and gain.

✓ Learn what your real caloric needs are and determine a diet plan that enables you to stay within the appropriate range.

✓ Accept the fact that weight loss takes time.

✓ Find and join a weight loss support group.

✓ Understand that to achieve long-term weight loss goals and maintain a healthier weight, you will have to make some permanent lifestyle changes that might not be easy to achieve.

4

Improving
Co-morbid Conditions

A study reported in the Cleveland Clinic Journal of Medicine in 2006 found that many co-morbid conditions are either greatly improved or resolved after bariatric surgery.[1]

Obesity-Related Health Problem	Percentage of Bariatric Surgery Patients
Asthma	82% improved or resolved
Cardiovascular Disease	82% risk reduction
Death	89% reduction in 5-year death rate
Depression	55% improved or resolved
Diabetes (Type 2)	83% resolved
Dyslipidemia hypercholesterolemia	63% resolved
Gastroesophageal reflux disease (GERD)	72 to 98% resolved
Hypertension (high blood pressure)	52 to 92% resolved
Metabolic Syndrome	80% resolved
Migraines	57% resolved

1   Stacy A Brethauer, Bipan Chand and Philip R Schauer. "Risks and benefits of bariatric surgery: current evidence." Cleveland Clinic Journal of Medicine 2006; 73(11):993-1007.

Obesity-Related Health Problem	Percentage of Bariatric Surgery Patients
Non-alcoholic fatty liver disease	90% improved steatosis 37% resolution of inflammation 20% reduction of fibrosis on repeat biopsy
Orthopedic problems or degenerative bone disease	41 to 70% resolved
Polycystic ovarian syndrome	78% resolution of hirsuitism 100% resolution of menstrual dysfunction
Pseudotumor cerebri	96% resolved
Sleep apnea	74 to 98% resolved
Stress urinary incontinence	44 to 88% resolved
Venous stasis disease	95% resolved

5

Eating Disorders

Most morbidly obese people have issues with food. It is likely that many of them have an eating disorder.

An *eating disorder* is characterized by abnormal eating habits that can involve either insufficient or excessive food intake that is detrimental to an individual's physical and emotional health.

Bariatric Surgery and Binge Eating Disorders

Unfortunately, bariatric surgery is neither a treatment nor a cure for binge eating disorders. Bariatric surgery can cause physical changes that can help you change the way you eat, but the emotional and psychological aspects of binge eating disorders are at least as important as the physical symptoms.

You can lose a significant amount of weight after bariatric surgery. However, continuing to binge will cause weight to be regained. Sometimes simply understanding the dynamics of why you binge can help to eliminate the problem; in other cases, you might need to talk to a psychologist or other counselor to gain some insight.

It is important to note that continuing to binge after bariatric surgery often leads to weight regain or weight loss that is significantly slower than it would be otherwise.

Since binge eating is a factor for many morbidly obese people, it is important to recognize any tendency to binge and to avoid it. Because night eating syndrome is a particularly efficient way to regain weight, any tendency for eating after dinner must be monitored for long-term success.

After bariatric surgery, your diet will seem to have become extremely important, and it is not unusual to harbor fear and anxiety where diet is concerned. The importance of joining and participating in a bariatric support group cannot be emphasized enough.

Binge Eating

Binge eating affects more people in the US than any other eating disorder, with bulemia and anorexia nervosa in second and third place respectively. Binge eating affects 3.5% of females and 2% of males in the US. [1]

It is not clear what causes eating disorders. There can be biological, psychological or environmental causes. Numerous studies have linked a genetic predisposition to eating disorders. Studies have also shown links between eating disorders and abused or neglected children, social isolation, cultural influence, parental influence, and peer pressure.

Interestingly, both binge eaters and bulemics indulge in binge eating. People with binge eating disorder do not display compensatory behavior, such as purging, the use of laxatives, or compulsive exercise. The binge eating is caused not by hunger but by emotional upset.

Night Eating Syndrome

Night Eating Syndrome is a newer form of binge eating disorder that is currently being studied. It is characterized by binge eating, but with specific behaviors: breakfast is skipped and the first meal is taken later in the day, and more than half of the daily calories are consumed after dinner. The excess calories frequently are carbohydrates. Since night eating syndrome tends to lead to weight gain, it was not surprising when one study reported in Newsweek magazine found that 28% of the participating bariatric patients suffered from night eating syndrome. People who suffer from this disorder often describe it as an uncontrollable desire to eat or an addiction to food.

---

1   PF Sullivan. "Mortality in anorexia nervosa." Biological Psychiatry Feb 2007 61(3)348-58:1073-1074. PMID 7793446.

Starvation Syndrome or Post-Surgical Eating Avoidance Disorder (PSEAD)

Post-bariatric surgical patients are often anxious or concerned about the process of starting to eat again after surgery. For the first few weeks, the diet is severely restricted and choices are limited. As time progresses, more foods are added to the diet and the prospect of having to make food decisions again must be considered. While post-surgery diets are almost always prescribed and relatively restricted, the ability to make food choices can be frightening.

Some bariatric patients harbor an inner fear that they will not eat enough after surgery. Patients subconsciously compare the amount of food being eaten after surgery with the often excessive quantity of food eaten for a number of years, and can feel deprived. They are unaware that the portions consumed after surgery are closer to a normal portion size than the excess quantity with which they were familiar.

While every post-bariatric patient has to ensure that they do not become malnourished, weight is lost in the first 12 to 18 months after surgery only if fewer calories are consumed than are needed to exist. This forces the body to use stored calories (in the form of stored fats in the body). The portions you consume after surgery are very close to normal portions for most foods – you will not starve if you continue to eat as directed by your bariatric team.

6

Diet and Lifestyle

A Doctor Discusses Food and Diet

My aunt Marlene sent this to me recently.

Q: Doctor, I've heard that cardiovascular exercise can prolong life. Is this true?

A: Your heart is only good for so many beats, and that's it. Don't waste them on exercise. Everything wears out eventually. Speeding up your heart won't make you live longer; it's like saying you extend the life of a car by driving it faster. Want to live longer? Take a nap.

Q: Should I cut down on meat and eat more fruits and vegetables?

A: You must grasp the concept of logistical efficiency. What does a cow eat? Hay and corn. And what are these? Vegetables. So steak is nothing more than an efficient mechanism for delivering vegetables to your system. Need grain? Eat chicken. Beef is a good source of field grass (green leafy vegetables).

Q: Should I reduce my alcohol intake?

A: No, not at all. Wine is made from fruit. Brandy is distilled wine, which means they take water out of the fruity bits so you get even more goodness that way. Beer is also made of grain.

Q: How can I calculate my body/fat ratio?

A: Well, if you have a body and you have fat, your ratio is one to one. If you have two bodies, your ratio is two to one.

Q: What are some of the advantages of participating in a regular exercise program?

A: I can't think of a single one, sorry. My philosophy is "no pain — good!"

Q: Aren't fried foods bad for you?

A: You aren't listening! Foods are fried these days in vegetable oil. In fact, they're permeated by it. How could getting more vegetables be bad for you?

Q: Will sit-ups prevent me from getting a little soft around the middle?

A: Definitely not. When you exercise muscle, it gets bigger. You should only be doing sit-ups if you want a bigger stomach.

Q: Is chocolate bad for me?

A: Are you crazy? Hellooooo! Cocoa beans! Another vegetable! It's the best feel-good food around.

Q: Is swimming good for your figure?

A: If swimming is good for your figure, explain whales to me.

Q: Is getting in shape important for my lifestyle?

A: Round is a shape!

Now that you're smiling (come on, admit it), let's get serious about the topic of your diet.

Diet and Lifestyle Changes

You absolutely must commit to making diet and lifestyle changes if you want to achieve a successful weight loss and avoid weight regain after bariatric surgery.

Some changes start before surgery. Your bariatric surgeon probably gave you a list of changes that were required before surgery, including:

✓ an initial weight loss of 5 to 10% of excess body weight, which reduces the amount of fat inside the abdomen, makes the internal organs more accessible and the surgery safer to perform

✓ an evaluation by a bariatric team, including dieticians and nutritionists, psychologists and other medical specialties as needed

✓ attendance at bariatric support group meetings for a specific amount of time before surgery, or for a specific number of meetings

✓ an evaluation of your weight loss history, including diet attempts, weight loss or regain and any previous surgeries

Patients who resist making lifestyle changes before their surgery often risk having their surgeon refuse to perform weight loss surgery. After all, you are the person who feeds you. If you won't even attempt losing weight without surgery, you are not a good candidate for long term weight loss or for maintaining the weight you lose after surgery.

Some of the long-term choices you must make include:

✓ controlling food portions for calorie reduction

✓ eating healthier foods

✓ eating foods that ensure good nutrition

✓ engaging in some physical activity that you enjoy

✓ participating in nutritional counseling to learn healthier ways of eating

✓ participating in counseling to deal with the emotional and mental aspects of obesity and weight loss surgery

✓ participating in bariatric support groups and online weight loss support forums

✓ setting goals and monitoring your success

✓ committing to long-term follow-up care with your bariatric surgical team

✓ making additional dietary and lifestyle changes as needed to prevent weight regain

Committing to long-term follow-up care with your bariatric team is extremely important and cannot be stressed enough. You will need regular tests every year or sometimes more frequently to monitor for nutritional deficiencies. This will continue for the rest of your life. Weight loss surgery has significant long-term effects, especially procedures that involve intestinal rerouting; many aspects are still unknown or not fully understood. A nutritional deficiency can develop at any time over the years. Your physician will test you regularly to check for vitamin and mineral deficiencies, protein malnutrition, anemia, bone disease, liver function and thyroid function.

As with many other aspects of weight loss surgery, how well you can tolerate various foods will be different. Another Roux-en-Y patient I know can eat sugars with impunity; if I eat more than 10 grams at a time, I develop stomach pain and nausea. Biliopancreatic diversion with duodenal switch patients vary widely in how well they can tolerate fats. The information in this chapter is intended as a guideline: if you have problems with specific foods, it can help you understand the anatomical and physiological reasons for the intolerance. After bariatric surgery, problems and food tolerance can change as time passes. The information presented here enables you to be aware of issues that others have encountered.

Lifestyle Changes After Bariatric Surgery

You can make lifestyle changes that will help to ensure successful weight loss after bariatric surgery. Failing to change some eating or behavioral habits can prevent long-term success.[1]

✓ Meal frequency — many overweight people tend to skip breakfast and then eat very large quantities in one or two meals per day. Since the capacity of the stomach is greatly reduced after surgery, you must learn to eat frequent small meals. Do not skip breakfast. Eat four to six very small nutritious meals throughout the day; do not eat after dinner.

✓ Eat less and slow down — you must learn to eat much slower than in the past. Eating too quickly can cause the stomach to fill up suddenly, which leads to nausea and vomiting. Many bariatric surgeons advise their patients to put their forks down for one full minute between bites, and to continue chewing the food while the fork is down. Constantly

---

1   Judy Dowd, "Nutrition Management After Gastric Bypass Surgery." Diabetes Spectrum, April 2005. Vol 18, Num 2, pp 82-84.

feeling nauseous or vomiting after eating can become a negative re-inforcement that can lead to malnutrition. It can take you 30 minutes to an hour to eat your meals and snacks.

✓ Chew your food more thoroughly and for a longer period. When food is swallowed, it should feel like baby food — mushy, with no chunks.

✓ When eating meat, you might need to concentrate on softer meats, including fish and poultry. Well-done meat, such as steak or roasts, can be difficult to digest; so can any meat that is fibrous.

✓ Do not drink fluids for 30 minutes before a meal, with a meal or for the 30 minutes after a meal. Be sure to drink in small sips. Your new smaller stomach might not be able to accommodate food and drink at the same time.

✓ Stay hydrated — because of the reduced size of the stomach, it can be difficult to drink enough fluids to stay well hydrated. Being de-hydrated causes additional problems, such as constipation and poor absorption of nutrients and medications. Do not rely on thirst as a trigger to drink. You should consume at least 64 ounces of fluids each day. Many foods, including soups, count as consumed fluids. Avoid sugary drinks or fruit beverages. Drink sugar-free drinks and always carry bottled water with you.

✓ Increase the number of servings of fruit, vegetables and whole grains — many people who are overweight do not consume enough serv-ings of fruits and vegetables. They also consume too many products made of refined flours. Fruits, vegetables and whole grains are good sources of fiber. Having enough fiber in the diet can prevent diarrhea or constipation, and also helps to reduce serum cholesterol.

✓ Avoid raw fruits or vegetables, except for bananas, and the skin of any cooked vegetables or fruit.

✓ Limit the amount of frying in fat and high-fat foods, especially fast food.

✓ Ensure adequate protein intake — bariatric surgeons recommend be-tween 60 and 80 grams per day of protein. Protein is required for nu-trition as well as wound healing after surgery. Some people are intolerant to many forms of protein, including red meat and poultry. Since many people are lactose intolerant, use altered milk products (ones that contain the enzyme lactase), reduce the quantity of milk products in your diet or eat thicker or processed diary foods like cheese or yogurt. Getting enough protein in the diet can be a problem. Visits with your nutritionist can help avoid problems with protein malnutrition.

✓ Avoid sweets – many bariatric patients were already addicted to sweets long before their surgery. Sugars can cause dumping syndrome in Roux-en-Y patients, especially from soda, juice drinks, milkshakes and ice cream. You must learn to eat healthier snacks, like nuts, trail mix or plain popcorn instead of sugary treats. Sugars in beverages are quickly absorbed and can cause discomfort. Avoid items with sugar that have more than 5 to 8 grams per serving size.

✓ Drinks with caffeine, like coffee and tea, can also cause problems. (Unfortunately, this also includes chocolate!)

✓ Take daily vitamin and mineral supplements — bariatric surgeries (other than lap band surgery) create malabsorption, which leads to nutritional deficiencies in calcium, iron and B-complex vitamins. You will take several supplements for the rest of your life. Blood tests taken during annual checkups with your bariatric surgeon can determine if you are developing nutritional deficiencies.

✓ Attend support group meetings — attending meetings provides moral support and encourages bariatric patients to socialize. Overweight people often isolate themselves. Other bariatric patients at support meetings have had experiences similar to yours; those who have achieved a successful weight loss can act as role models for patients who are still going through the process.

✓ Exercise — most obese people do not get enough exercise. While even couch potatoes can lose weight after bariatric surgery, the excess weight will return if your eating habits do not change or if you do not move more. Exercise also helps reduce the amount of sagging skin and flaccid muscles that can require plastic surgery after significant weight loss.

The Secret of Successful Weight Loss

The single most important change you can make after surgery is to follow your bariatric surgeon's instructions.

In a new survey of 282 bariatric surgeons and 409 patients who underwent gastric banding or gastric bypass in the previous one to five years, those patients who heeded their doctor's advice following surgery lost about 35 percent more weight than those who did not take their doctor's advice as seriously or as literally. Those who listened were also more likely to keep the weight off. The survey findings were released at the 25th annual meeting of the American Society for Metabolic and Bariatric Surgery in Washington, D.C. in June, 2008.

The survey also found that patients who underwent gastric band surgery had significantly better long-term results than other gastric band patients. These patients had more frequent adjustments to their gastric band, which more effectively controlled their diet.

Achieving and Maintaining the Ideal Weight

While bariatric surgery has many beneficial effects, most people seek the surgery to reduce their body weight. About one third of the American population is seriously or morbidly obese. It is estimated that about two thirds of Americans are overweight. There is a strong genetic tendency to be overweight; if your parents and grandparents were overweight, chances are higher that you will be too. Our environment also contributes to obesity. Physical activity is not often required in our culture, and foods that cost the least have the most calories and fewest nutrients. While most people are aware of how nutrition works, they do not follow good eating habits.

Recent studies show significant increases in obesity in the Southeastern United States, but obesity in general is increasing across the country.

Weight loss after bariatric surgery is relatively simple to achieve. The restrictive surgeries discourage overeating. The malabsorptive surgeries enable much of the food that is consumed to pass through the digestive tract without extracting all of its calories. The surgeries that are both restrictive and malabsorptive perform both functions, with greater weight loss achieved more quickly.

It should be noted, however, that over time, the final results become more similar.

There are several weight management issues to consider as you decide to have bariatric surgery. Weight management and control is a lifelong task; it is not achieved simply because you had bariatric surgery. You will always have to keep your weight in mind and take specific steps each day to maintain it.

Determining a Baseline

Before your weight loss surgery, most bariatric surgeons require a battery of tests and evaluations that are designed to help determine the chances of success in losing excess weight and maintaining a healthier weight. A multidisciplinary team is assembled, consisting of the bariatric surgeon, a nutritionist and a psychologist; others might be included as determined by the surgeon.

This screening process includes a thorough medical evaluation, a psychological evaluation, nutritional counseling and education about the bariatric surgery and what to expect, both shortly after surgery and over a long time period. Psychologists review the patient's past history for signs of depression, among other conditions, which can short-circuit long–term success. A person's mood and eating habits are closely related.

Weight loss surgeries such as Roux-en-Y and biliopancreatic diversion with duodenal switch, which have both restrictive and malabsorptive components, cause a rapid weight loss during the twelve to eighteen months following surgery. Procedures like gastric band surgery, which are only restrictive, result in a slower weight loss; although similar results to Roux-en-Y and biliopancreatic diversion with duodenal switch surgeries are experienced, the same results typically take about twice as long — nearly 3 years in many cases.

With any weight loss surgery, weight loss is achieved mostly in the early period after surgery, after which time the body begins to adjust and weight loss slows. About 20% of all weight loss patients experience either an inadequate weight loss or regain a significant amount of weight.

Eating patterns after surgery can increase weight loss or sabotage it. These include:

✓ frequent snacking or grazing

✓ consuming high calorie foods

✓ binge eating or night eating syndrome

✓ poor food choices, such as consuming too many high-calorie liquids (milkshakes, fruit juices)

✓ oversized portions

These behaviors make it possible to consume a large amount of calories despite the surgically-reduced capacity of the stomach.

Thankfully, developing eating disorders after surgery is not likely. Failure to control eating leads to weight gain, but only a small number of patients develop this behavior who did not display signs of having the problem before surgery.

A study completed in 2004 proposed a new diagnosis for *post surgical eating avoidance disorder* (PSEAD), which is characterized by an eating disorder and anxiety symptoms that occur at the same time after bariatric surgery. This disorder has also been called starvation syndrome.

Patients who exhibited pre-surgical eating disorders should continue to seek counseling and follow-up after their bariatric surgery, since they have a slightly elevated risk of further developing eating disorders after surgery.

Early Weight Loss

Bariatric surgery has been available for more than 50 years. Over time, many studies have been completed that purport to show the definitive amount of weight lost after various forms of weight loss surgery. Different studies show varying rates of success, depending on when and where the study was done, the time span and the end results. Groups of patients varied widely. Some studies used control groups to obtain averages or ratios, while other studies included only bariatric patients.

As expected, the results showed a wide range of weight loss success.

The interesting fact is that there were many successful weight losses in a population in which the history of weight loss was difficult or nearly impossible. People who had tried every diet plan in the world were suddenly thinner and staying that way.

And, as an additional reward, dangerous co–morbid conditions were either eliminated or improved!

✓ Roux-en-Y patients lose 50-60% of excess weight in 2 years

✓ Biliopancreatic Diversion with Duodenal Switch patients lose 70% of current weight or 35% of BMI over 18 months

✓ Gastric band patients lose 60% of weight after 2 years

Overcoming a Weight Plateau

After weight loss surgery, you lose weight rapidly at first, but as time passes, the weight loss becomes more gradual. In many cases, weight begins to stabilize around twelve to eighteen months following surgery, depending on which procedure was used; with gastric band surgery, weight loss can continue slowly for two to three years.

Weight loss during this period does not follow a steady pattern; it is erratic with periods of significant weight loss followed by periods with little or no weight loss. When weight loss slows, patients wonder whether they are doing something wrong or if the surgical procedure was a failure.

Weight loss is not just about the loss of fat cells. Both men and women can retain excess fluid for various reasons, giving the impression that no weight was lost. For this reason, it is important to stay hydrated after surgery.

Other reasons can result in weight loss plateaus:

✓ The amount of food moving through the gastrointestinal tract adds to body weight.

✓ If you are exercising more, you might be gaining muscle mass, which is less bulky than fat but weighs more.

✓ Changes in eating habits can drastically affect weight loss rates. Eating too many meals a day or grazing between meals can slow weight loss.

✓ The composition of foods in the diet can affect weight loss. If weight loss slows, eat more protein and less carbohydrates.

✓ Women who are menstruating can retain a significant amount of fluid temporarily, which normally disappears when their cycle is complete.

✓ A change in the amount or frequency of exercise can alter the metabolism, resulting in more or less weight loss at different times.

After malabsorptive surgery like Roux-en-Y and biliopancreatic diversion with duodenal switch surgeries, the body adjusts over time and begins to better absorb nutrients (and calories) from the diet, which can reduce weight loss. After the body adapts to the anatomical changes, it processes fats and carbohydrates more efficiently. To counteract this effect, eat more protein and fewer fats and carbohydrates.

Avoid the tendency to drink liquids with meals. Liquids can help move the contents of the stomach into the gastrointestinal tract, increasing absorption. As food is moved out of the stomach pouch, it delays the sensation of feeling full, causing further overeating. An emptied stomach also allows the ingestion of larger portions.

Remember, nobody promises a steady weight loss after bariatric surgery. Reaching weight plateaus is a normal part of the weight loss process. If it happens, first examine your eating habits to see if you are short-circuiting your own efforts in some way. If not, accept the plateau as a signal that your body is adjusting to its anatomical changes and that weight loss will happen as long as you continue to follow the post-surgical plan set out for you by your bariatric team.

Weight Gain

About 20% of all weight loss surgery patients report regaining a significant amount of weight over a five year period after losing it successfully in the first twelve to eighteen months following surgery. That amounts to one patient in five.

People who had malabsorptive weight loss surgery, including Roux-en-Y and biliopancreatic diversion with duodenal switch surgeries, usually gain back about 8 to 10% of the pounds they lost. Those who had restrictive surgeries usually gain back slightly less weight. However, over the long term, malabsorptive procedures resulted in greater total weight loss than restrictive procedures. Short-term studies indicate that the rates become similar at about five years after surgery. Studies of how patients fare over longer time periods are currently underway, but results will not be available for several years.

You can regain weight regardless of the type of procedure you had.

It must be emphasized that weight loss surgery is only a tool. If you keep pushing too much food or the wrong types of food through that pie hole, it's a fact that you'll gain weight.

Minimizing Weight Gain After Bariatric Surgery

After losing weight and reaching your goal, it is important to maintain your weight.

After fifty years of watching one of my sisters, I finally decided to follow her method, which has kept her weight at about the same as when she graduated high school. Her secret could not be more simple; it has only two steps that are easy to follow.

1   Weigh yourself every day.

2   If you gain more than five pounds, immediately cut back on food intake and, if necessary, increase exercise, until the extra five pounds are gone.

After reaching goal weight on the Optifast diet two decades ago, I watched as the scales showed a very gradual but steady increase in my weight. I went from "I've only put on an extra twenty pounds, so I'm still close to my goal weight" to "where did those fifty pounds come from?" I'll admit to being a procrastinator, but where health and vitality are concerned, nobody can afford not to be diligent about weight regain.

The reason for weighing yourself every day is that people who were formerly obese can gain weight very quickly by going back to unhealthy eating habits or becoming lax with their attempts at exercise. If you have a restrictive or malabsorptive weight loss surgery, it is nearly impossible to regain pounds in a day or two. However, by not paying attention over the course of a week, you stand a much greater chance for adding five pounds or more.

Some weight loss patients achieve their goal weight and find that they look too thin or emaciated, so they deliberately regain five or ten pounds. Weight loss surgery is strenuous on the body, so it is not uncommon to get to goal weight and look a bit unhealthy. As time passes, your body will adapt to the anatomical changes and if you maintain your goal weight, you will begin to look healthier. It is also normal to get to goal weight and regain a few pounds without trying to do it deliberately.

There are some potential pitfalls that must be addressed early on.

✓ **Stop binge eating and night eating before your weight loss surgery.** People who binge tend to lose less weight after surgery.

✓ **Lose as much weight as possible before surgery.** The lower your body mass index, the more weight you'll lose and your lower weight will be easier to maintain. One study showed that people with a BMI between 35 and 39.9 were much more likely than those with a BMI higher than 40 to keep off at least half of their excess weight ten years after surgery.

✓ **Address alcohol and drug abuse problems, if you have them, before surgery.** Both issues can cause weight gain. Both lead to increased complications from bariatric surgery. The psychological interview that you are required to attend before surgery is scheduled can reveal this problem if it exists.

✓ **Follow your bariatric surgeon's advice explicitly.** Bariatric doctors require follow-up visits on a regular basis, and their patients tend to lose more weight and keep it off more than patients who abandoned their doctors after their surgery. Seeing your bariatric surgeon regularly is also more likely to discover potential problems earlier.

✓ **Join and participate in a good bariatric support group.** Patients who join and continue to interact with a support group maintain a 10% lower body mass index than those who do not.

✓ **Immediately address food issues if you experience them after surgery.** If you experience increasing food urges, depression or other emotional problems, discuss them with your bariatric surgeon. People who experience these issues but don't address them usually regain more weight.

✓ **Continue to get nutritional counseling.** After a period of time passes and weight is lost, it becomes easy to slip into old habits. This causes weight gain. Patients who continue to follow-up with nutritionists or dieticians have better long-term weight loss.

Reversing Weight Gain With Additional Surgery

Before considering additional surgery to reverse weight gain after bariatric surgery, your surgeon will require you to adhere to a diet and exercise regimen.

If your stomach pouch has stretched and is no longer restrictive enough, there are some surgical remedies that can help. Note that revisional surgery carries additional risks and it is more difficult than the original bariatric surgery because of the scar tissue that has formed.

- ✓ **Endoscopic injection of a sclerosant (sodium morrhuate) to shrink the stomach.** An injection of sodium morrhuate is injected two or three times during an endoscopic procedure. Several injections are usually necessary to shrink the stomach enough. One study showed that 64% of patients who had this surgery lost 75% of the weight they regained. One complication is *stomal stenosis*, a shrinkage that requires the stomach to be stretched again using a special balloon.

- ✓ **Restorative obesity surgery, endoluminal (ROSE) technique.** This procedure is also performed endoscopically. It places tissue anchors to reduce stomach size. Several studies have shown it to be effective in reducing the size of the stomach and causing weight loss in Roux-en-Y patients. One analysis showed that 88% of patients stopped regaining weight and that 96% of patients had lost 18% of their excess weight six months after the procedure.

- ✓ **Altering the anastomosis.** The anastomosis is the opening between the stomach pouch and the intestinal tract. It can stretch after surgery. This procedure tightens the opening and increases the restriction.

- ✓ **Non-adjustable silicone ring.** A more invasive procedure, this requires placement of a silicone ring around the stomach pouch. The ring is not adjustable. It has been shown to increase the percentage of excess weight loss by around 23%.

Insufficient Weight Loss

A similar problem is encountered by weight loss patients who never lose a significant amount of their excess weight.

This problem is most frequently caused by continuing to ingest too many calories. Snacking or grazing between meals is often to blame. Eating high-calorie foods contributes to the problem, as does simply eating too much.

The restrictive portion of the surgery might not have been sufficient enough to truly reduce calorie intake. People who continue to overeat lose weight more slowly, and slower weight loss can lead the patient to believe that the surgery was not successful. Those who lose weight more slowly than anticipated can subconsciously sabotage their efforts.

If you had gastric band surgery, your bariatric surgeon can tighten the band to increase the restriction. Other forms of surgery, like Roux-en-Y and biliopancreatic diversion with duodenal switch surgeries might need revisional surgery if the stomach pouch is truly too large or has stretched. Revisional surgery has its own complications, one of which involves the scar tissue from the previous surgery.

The anastomosis also might have stretched, increasing the amount of food that can pass through it. Revisional surgery can reduce the size of the anastomosis.

If you achieve a weight loss rate that is significantly lower statistically than should be expected, your bariatric surgeon might request you to see a nutritionist to check your diet, or to see a psychologist. Emotional issues often cause slower weight loss, including lack of support from family or friends or not attending a bariatric support group.

A very small percentage of people never lose weight as quickly as they think they should. The secret to long–term weight loss success is to stay on your bariatric diet program and increase, if possible, your exercise levels. Making a long-term commitment to weight loss is a lifelong process.

Developing New Diet and Eating Habits

Before you had your bariatric surgery, your bariatric surgeon required you to begin a weight-loss regimen and lose a portion of your excess weight. Many health insurance providers require that you go through a medically supervised weight loss program before they approve your surgery. This diet was probably high protein and low carbohydrate with plenty of fluids.

The changes that were made to your digestive system during surgery require some changes in your diet and eating habits. Here are some recommendations:

✓ Eat healthy foods. For more information, see "What Are Healthy Foods?" on page 61.

✓ Eat four to six very small meals each day.

✓ Eat meals at planned times.

✓ Do not skip breakfast. Include proteins in your breakfast foods.

✓ Chew food slowly and completely. Do not swallow large chunks of food. If you find it difficult to eat more slowly, put your fork down between bites and leave it on the table for one full minute. During that time, continue to chew your food.

✓ Drink fluids at times other than when you are eating. Do not drink for the 30 minutes before a meal, or for 60 minutes afterwards. Drinking while eating causes the food to pass too quickly from the stomach. It also makes you feel full faster, which causes you to eat less, which in turn can result in malnutrition. However, drink often during the rest of the day to keep the digestive tract active and flowing. Additional fluids do not cause diarrhea.

✓ Drink at least 8 cups (that's 64 ounces or half a gallon) of fluids each day.

✓ Fluids should not contain any calories, or be very low calorie. Diet frozen juice bars can help fulfill your fluid requirements. Avoid fruit juices, which are high in calories and carbohydrates. Fizzy (carbonated) drinks can cause excess gas and bloating.

✓ Avoid very hot or very cold foods.

✓ Avoid foods high in sugars and fats, like fruit drinks, non-diet sodas, milkshakes or high calorie nutritional supplements. These foods can cause dumping syndrome if you had Roux-en-Y surgery, insufficient weight loss or weight regain.

✓ Eat proteins with every meal. High protein foods include egg whites, lean meats, beans, and dairy products.

✓ Eat proteins first to ensure adequate intake. The recommended long-term protein intake is usually between 60 and 80 grams per day. Pay careful attention to the quantity of fats that often coexist with proteins.

✓ Increase the number of servings of fruits, vegetables and whole grains. These foods contain fiber, which prevents constipation and diarrhea.

✓ Reduce the quantity of starches, which are often trigger foods for overweight people who might develop an intolerance for starches. While the body needs carbohydrates, eat healthier carbohydrates instead, like fruits and vegetables, and in moderation. Use whole grain breads, brown rice and whole grain pastas when you want to include a starch with the meal.

✓ Take daily vitamin and mineral supplements in quantities higher than recommended for the normal (that is, those who have not had bariatric surgery) population. You will probably not get enough nutrition from the smaller meals you consume.

✓ Patients who have had malabsorptive surgeries like Roux-en-Y and biliopancreatic diversion with duodenal switch must be monitored for iron, calcium and B-complex vitamin deficiencies. Annual blood tests performed during your annual follow-up appointment with your bariatric surgeon will monitor you for these deficiencies.

✓ Avoid alcohol. It is absorbed and metabolized much more quickly after surgery, causing unexpected intoxication even after smaller amounts than you might have consumed before surgery. Alcohol can cause ulcers in the stomach and intestines.

✓ Avoid snacks. Frequent snacking (grazing) can cause weight gain.

✓ Measure foods with a small kitchen scale. Don't estimate quantity — it doesn't usually work well. Overweight people tend to underestimate their calorie content per meal by as much as 25%.

✓ Use small plates and small utensils. Using regular sized plates makes the smaller portion sizes look even tinier.

✓ Avoid watching TV, especially while eating. Research shows that the more you watch, the more likely you'll be to get away from your diet.

If you have a DVR, record the shows you like and fast-forward through the commercials.

✓ Avoid fast food restaurants. Even so-called "healthy foods" sold at fast food restaurants tend to have significantly more fat and calories than those prepared at home. If a meal in a restaurant cannot be avoided, stick to salads with small portions of dressing and calorie-free beverages.

✓ If your stomach feels irritated or upset, switch to soft foods for the next meal or two, and increase your fluid intake.

Resources for Preparing Bariatric Meals

One of the secrets of learning to eat well after bariatric surgery is to learn how to prepare your food so that it retains its healthy aspects and tastes good too.

There are several cookbooks for post-bariatric surgery patients that can help.

Recipes for Life After Weight Loss Surgery: Delicious Dishes for Nourishing the New You, by Margaret M. Furtado and Lynette Schultz. Fairwinds Press, Healthy Living Cookbooks, Feb 2007. 240 pgs. ISBN 978-1592332267.

Cooking for Weight Loss Surgery Patients, by Dick Stucki. Bonneville Publishing, 200 pgs, Feb 2005. ISBN 978-0925838148.

The Complete Idiot's Guide to Eating Well After Weight Loss Surgery, by Margaret Furtado and Joseph Ewing. Alpha Publications, Dec 2009. 384 pgs. Alpha, Dec 2009. 384 pgs. ISBN 978-1592579518.

Eating Well After Weight Loss Surgery: Over 140 Delicious Low Fat High-Protein Recipes to Enjoy in the Weeks, Months and Years After Surgery, by Patt Levine, Michele Bontempo-Saray, William B. Inabnet, and Meredith Urban-Skuros. Da Capo Press, July 2004. 193 pgs. ISBN 978-1569244531.

There are other cookbooks that can help you prepare foods suitable for a bariatric diet. Since a large volume of information is readily available, including recipes here is beyond the scope of this book.

You can do an Internet search to find additional resources, or search on Amazon.com for "weight loss cookbooks" or "weight control cookbooks." Many bariatric websites also provide appropriate recipes.

Those who attend bariatric support groups will be inundated with recipes and cooking tips from people who use them in everyday life.

If you don't know how to cook, there are many small companies that prepare complete meals for you and deliver them to you for a reasonable price. In many cities, you can also hire private chefs to prepare meals and freeze them for later use. These companies and chefs can take into account any dietary restrictions you have and find creative ways to ensure you have nutritious meals to eat.

What Are Healthy Foods?

Immediately after your surgery, your surgical team tells you to eat healthy foods. How do you know what foods are healthy?

Here is an acronym that has proved useful: **FOG.**

✓ **Farm** — any foods raised on a farm (dairy products, eggs, and poultry)

✓ **Ocean** — any food that comes from the ocean (fish, shellfish)

✓ **Ground** — anything grown in the ground (fruits, vegetables, nuts, whole grains)

Note that these foods are the ones sold along the outside edges of the grocery store. Avoid the center aisles, where foods tend to be more processed or have more additives. Look for those foods that are unadulterated and in their natural state: chicken breasts, for example, instead of breaded chicken tenders, or fresh broccoli instead of frozen broccoli with cheese sauce.

An unhealthy food is any food that's significantly modified by humans. Read the label. If there are more than six ingredients, ingredients created or manufactured in a laboratory, or any ingredients that you can't pronounce, don't buy it.

After buying healthy food, be sure to prepare it in a healthy way.

✓ When cooking, bake, grill, poach or broil — avoid frying because it tends to toughen proteins and can also add fats and their calories to your foods.

✓ Use chicken or vegetable broth instead of oil.

✓ Use skim milk instead of whole milk.

✓ Use spices or lemon juice to add flavor instead of olive oil or butter.

✓ Use applesauce or yogurt in place of oil in recipes.

After bariatric surgery, many people report that eating in a more healthy way is preferable to their old eating habits. It is common to be turned off by foods that you previously enjoyed before surgery.

One good resource is the Bariatric Surgery Nutritional Guidelines from the American Society of Metabolic and Bariatric Surgery (ASMBA). The Guidelines are updated regularly. You can find a downloadable PDF version at:

        http://www.asmbs.org/Newsite07/resources/bgs_final.pdf

What About Portion Sizes?

During your bariatric surgery, your surgeon creates a smaller stomach pouch. This is not an absolutely scientific procedure: surgeons use anatomical reference points within each patient to determine the size of the stomach pouch. Since each person's body is different, no two bariatric patients have exactly the same size stomach pouch.

However, in general, your new pouch should be able to hold about one cup of food. That's about 4 ounces per meal. Gastric band patients who can consume a larger quantity probably need to have the gastric band tightened.

While your meal portions are considerably smaller than they used to be, you might also have to eat less than the restricted portion size. You must learn to stop eating just before you begin to feel full. In the past, most overweight people continue to consume food past the point of mild discomfort. If you did that routinely before your bariatric surgery, you will find that mealtimes become a problem because you will begin to associate eating with discomfort.

Continuing to eat beyond the point of feeling full causes vomiting, diarrhea, constipation or difficulty swallowing. Overeating even small amounts will cause your stomach to stretch, leading to insufficient weight loss or weight regain.

Pay attention to the quantity of food you can eat at each meal without feeling full. Weigh the food before you start to eat, and weigh any remaining food when you stop eating — before feeling full. Subtract the remaining amount from the starting amount; the difference is the weight of the portion size that you can enjoy.

Different foods weigh differently, depending on how bulky or dense the food item is. Use a kitchen scale to weigh several types of food a few times to get a basis from which to work.

When in doubt, remember that it is better to leave some food on the plate, uneaten, rather than consuming it all and feeling uncomfortable afterwards!

Additionally, you can learn to eat smaller portion sizes by putting your food on smaller plates. The mind is easily tricked into thinking that a "plate full of food" is the same quantity as it was before surgery. I found this trick works well. I now eat almost everything from luncheon-sized plates, rather than the much larger dinner plates. I also have my servings of soup in smaller dessert dishes rather than the larger soup bowls.

You should also try to eat smaller forkfuls of food. I cut into smaller portions any food that I would have eaten in large chunks before surgery.

If you eat more slowly, you will also avoid sitting with an empty plate at the table with family or friends who are still eating. Pace your eating so that everyone at the table finishes at about the same time. Since you will be eating less food, you'll have to eat more slowly to accomplish this.

What Not To Eat

After bariatric surgery, there is a long list of foods that you cannot eat. Common foods can upset your digestive system causing problems such as difficulty swallowing, vomiting, diarrhea or constipation.

As your body becomes used to the changes that were made during surgery, you might be able to eat some of these foods in larger quantities. Others, however, will continue to bother you consistently over time. As time passes, you can continue to try these foods, eating smaller quantities than normal, or you might need to give up that food altogether.

Here are some foods that might be have to be eliminated or eaten less frequently or in smaller amounts, depending on your body and the type of surgery you chose:

✓ carbonated beverages

✓ soft or doughy bread

✓ pasta

✓ tough or dry red meat

✓ nuts

✓ popcorn

✓ fibrous foods

✓ coffee

✓ alcohol

Eliminate the following foods from your diet forever:

✓ sugar, foods containing sugars, and concentrated sweets

✓ fruit juice

✓ high saturated fat

✓ fried foods

Signs of Problems With Bariatric Eating

Pay attention to these symptoms while learning how to eat after bariatric surgery:

✓ **Feeling full.** Before bariatric surgery, most people eat until they feel full. After the surgery, you need to avoid the sensation of feeling full, since that point literally can be only another bite from becoming nauseous. You feel full when your stomach is full — but if you're still eating, additional food will be on its way down the esophagus, and this food has not yet reached the stomach or caused you to feel satisfied. When it does all finally move into the stomach, it can be considerably too much food.

✓ **Discomfort in the chest, including chest pain or pressure.** Take note of what foods you ate, and how much you ate before you noticed the discomfort. You can reduce portion sizes or avoid some foods altogether. If the feeling continues, discuss this problem with your bariatric surgeon immediately.

✓ **Nausea or vomiting.** If this happens quickly and then passes, look at the foods you ate recently. It can be caused by something you ate. Being dehydrated also causes nausea and vomiting, so you might need to increase the amount of fluids you drink each day.

✓ **Vomiting that does not stop, or abdominal pain.** Contact your surgeon immediately. These symptoms can be caused by surgical complications or intestinal hernia. They must be resolved quickly.

✓ **Gas, bloating or cramping.** These symptoms are almost always caused by the foods you eat. You can reduce the quantity or frequency of these foods, or avoid them completely. You can also try to prepare the food in a different way. For example, fried chicken might not agree with you, but poached or broiled chicken might be acceptable instead.

Emotional Eating and Bariatric Surgery

Any time you eat for reasons other than satisfying your body's nutritional needs, you are eating emotionally.

Research has shown that bariatric surgery has an equally positive impact on weight loss and eating behavior for both high and low emotional eaters.[2]

In addition, having an eating disorder before surgery has no relationship to the success of the surgery.[3]

2   S Fischer, E Chen, S Katterman, M Roerhig, L Bochierri-Ricciardi, D Munoz, M Dymek-Valentine, J Alverdy, D le Grange. "Emotional Eating in a Morbidly Obese Bariatric Surgery-Seeking Population." Obesity Surgery Journal. June 2007. Vol 17, Num 6, pgs 778-784.

3   JF Kinzl, M Schrattenecker, C Traweger, M Mattesich, M Fiala, W Biebl. "Psychosocial Predictors of Weight Loss after Bariatric Surgery." Obesity Surgery Journal. December 2006. Vol 16, Num 12, pgs 1609-1614.

The good news is that there is a good chance that your cravings will go away entirely or be reduced to a controllable level after bariatric surgery.

Keep a Food Journal

In the support group I attended before my weight-loss surgery there was a small group of people who sat apart and resisted any new idea that would change their life. We were told to keep food journals. The most outspoken members of that group ridiculed the idea, said it would not work, and refused to keep the journal.

After weight-loss surgery, the people in the support group who had the most problem keeping off the weight they lost or losing weight in general were the same people who has resisted keeping a food journal.

Use the food journal to plan and record your meals. You can keep a hard copy journal using paper and pen, or use an online food journal. In either case take a printed copy of your journal with you to the grocery store (or print out your list) and only buy the foods that you plan.

You can also use the journal to set your goals and record progress.

Your food journal does not need to be kept with meticulous detail. Simply jotting down the foods you ate and the quantity eaten is enough to be useful in determining trends and problem areas.

Your food journal contains notes that you might find helpful and are included only for yourself. It is not a literary work, and does not have to be perfect or formatted nicely for others to read. Neatness does not count, nor does how thorough it is. It's better to jot down a few notes that are meaningful to you than to insist on writing perfect prose that you find tedious to do and ultimately abandon. This journal is for you.

Eating Away From Home After Bariatric Surgery

Eating away from home can be problematic for weight loss surgery patients.

When you prepare your own meals at home, you can control the ingredients, the method of cooking, and the portion sizes. When you eat out – whether in restaurants or other people's homes — you lose control of these areas.

You might also find that restaurant food contains too much salt. The quantity of salt in a post-bariatric diet influences fluid retention; this is often compounded for many people who had heart and circulatory issues before their surgery.

Here are some tips for eating away from home:

✓ Ask for a child's portion or a senior portion. The amount of food on the plate reflects the portion size, not the age of the patron. If the restaurant fusses about the issue, you can tell them you had weight loss surgery and cannot eat a regular portion. If the wait staff refuses to be reasonable, eat somewhere else where your patronage is better appreciated.

✓ Take half of your dinner home in a doggie bag. One of the great joys in my life is that I now eat two restaurant meals for the price of one: the first half at the restaurant, and the second portion the next day.

✓ Ask the server to have your meal prepared in a specific way. You can request that proteins are broiled or baked instead of fried.

✓ Many restaurants allow you to order an item and split it between two people. This is an easy way to control portion size and still enjoy eating out.

✓ Don't drink before you eat. Non-alcoholic beverages are filling; alcoholic beverages are not well tolerated, and achieving higher levels of intoxication more quickly than before surgery can make you feel nauseous.

✓ Eat an appetizer instead of a main course. Besides being less expensive, the portion size is smaller and often ideal for weight loss surgery patients.

✓ Avoid soups and salads. Both tend to make you feel full quickly. If you plan to eat an entree and still crave soup or a salad, choose a small portion of soup, eat it slowly, and ask the server to take some time before delivering the rest of your meal. Your stomach can process soup faster than salad, freeing some space for your entree.

✓ Avoid large meals. These are called table d'hote (host's table), prix fixe (fixed price), plat du jour (dish of the day), blue plate specials or set menu meals, in which multi-course meals with only a few choices are charged at a fixed price. It often includes a starter, main dish, bread, drink, and choice of coffee or dessert. This type of meal is great for lumberjacks and weight lifters, but weight loss surgery patients cannot possibly eat even a portion of this spread. Order a la carte from the menu instead and order only the amount of food you know you can eat.

✓ Avoid buffet or "all you can eat" restaurants, for the same reason.

✓ Avoid sports bars, nightclubs, or any place where you are distracted while you eat. You eat less if you pay attention while consuming the food.

While it is easier to adapt restaurant meals to your new dietary lifestyle, eating in friends' homes is also possible. Your friends will probably know that you have had bariatric surgery; most people attempt to be supportive and will do what they can to accommodate your new diet. If you don't want to discuss your weight loss surgery, you can say you have food allergies that prevent you from eating certain types of foods. You can discuss your dietary needs and restrictions beforehand so that they are aware of any issues you might have with what they plan to serve.

If your host has planned a specific menu of foods that you cannot have, decline the invitation and plan to join them at another time when the food choices will be different. The majority of your friends will be understanding and supportive; those who are not are probably not worth socializing with anyway!

7

Exercise

Most people believe that overweight people just do not exercise enough, if they exercise at all. In many cases, this is completely unfounded. Many obese people are physically active, and many are more active than thinner folks.

The act of walking, working or exercising while carrying a hundred or more extra pounds certainly qualifies as exercise!

While the amount of exercise you take does not determine your weight, it is an important consideration when losing weight and attempting to maintain a weight loss.

If you eat normally and don't move much, you will probably tend to gain weight, regardless of whether you are already overweight or underweight.

After massive weight loss, how you look depends on many factors; muscle tone and activity levels play an important part in regaining a body shape that is pleasing and proportional.

Exercising has a negative connotation, especially among the obese, but everyone would like to be active and vital. It might be more appropriate to call this an *activity plan*. Your activity plan does not have to include weight lifting, running or any traditional "exercise." You simply have to increase the amount of physical activity, and that can include doing many pleasurable things, like walking or dancing.

An exercise plan should begin before surgery and resume as soon as your bariatric surgeon allows after surgery.

Increasing your activity level can help you:

✓ increase energy levels

✓ tone muscles

✓ boost metabolism

✓ tone the muscles and skin

✓ decrease cardiac disease and lower blood pressure

✓ improve your outlook on life

Adding 30 minutes each day of physical activity is enough to realize a benefit. The increased activities can be anything other than your normal activities for the day. Normal activities include working, housekeeping or yard chores. Any activity that you would not have had to do to get through the day qualifies as an added activity.

Walking instead of driving or riding is the single activity that has the most benefit. If you regularly take a bus, walk down the street to the next stop and get on there instead of the stop closest to your door. If you drive, look for a space to park as far as possible from your destination. If you go to the bank, park the car as far from the door as possible and walk inside instead of using the drive-up window. If you frequent stores and shops in your neighborhood, walk there instead of driving or taking public transportation. Climb the stairs instead of taking the elevator.

You can search the Internet for bariatric exercise programs that can guide your activity plan. The Bariatric Choice website has a 12-point program that gradually increases in intensity and provides specific exercises that anyone can perform.

http://www.bariatricchoice.com/exercise-for-bariatric-gastric-bypass-surgery-patients.aspx

Start Slowly

If you have not exercised in a long time — this is the norm for people who are overweight — it is important to start slowly. It is easy to get caught up in the enthusiasm of a new weight loss program, especially one that can be expected to produce excellent results for most people. However, if you have been very sedentary, it is unwise to stress your muscles (and bones, which are also affected by exercise) too much at the start of a new exercise regime.

Start with stretching exercises for the first few days, and do not do much more than stretching. Give your body a chance to acclimate itself to being in motion again. This reduces the chance for injury. If your muscles tense up or feel strained, stop doing what you're doing. Go for a walk instead.

After a few days, your muscles will no longer become tense when you start moving vigorously. Add a simple movement or two and do only a few repetitions. Do not repeat any exercise if it becomes painful or difficult.

As time progresses, you will easily be able to include additional exercises and to tolerate them for longer periods.

It is often helpful to alternate the types of exercise you do. You can walk, ride a bicycle, dance, go bowling, or go to the gym for weight training or Pilates classes; varying the kinds of exercise you do helps avoid boredom and gives muscles a chance to rest and recuperate. Each activity uses different muscles, so varying the types of exercise you take helps strengthen the entire body.

Make an Activity Plan

An extensive exercise plan is beyond the scope of this book. There are Internet resources to help you understand what is involved, along with printed books and the knowledge of personal trainers and fitness center employees. Your exercise plan must be set up to address your specific needs. Take the time and effort to prepare an effective activity plan that will help you achieve your weight loss goals.

Join a Fitness Center

Even people who enjoy exercising need motivation. Joining a fitness center can help. It is easier to skip exercise sessions if you work alone. At a fitness center, you will begin to see familiar faces, and those people can form a support team for your exercise activity.

When I lost weight, a friend and I joined a fitness center and instead of eating at lunch hour, we went to the center and walked on the track for an hour. At first, we struggled to get around the track a single time. Within a month, we were doing multiple laps, and by the end of the fourth month, we were walking 5 miles a day — and enjoying it. Several people exercised at the same time each day, and we got to know them as we walked past on the track. One weight lifter was very supportive, and when my friend wasn't able to walk with me, he would stop what he was doing and join me so that I would stay motivated. Needless to say, we became friends, thanks to his incredible support. Before I joined, I was afraid that people would snicker at me, the fat guy, but instead I discovered a number of people who were supportive and encouraging as I lost weight. I felt that if I wasn't successful, I would be letting all of them down. That additional motivation helped me overcome the discouragement of a couple of weight plateaus.

Sadly, Mike VanKleek, my weight lifter friend, did not live long enough to see me reach my goal weight. He died at age 40 of a brain hemorrhage, possibly from lifting too much weight. Ironically, he was in perfect physical condition. However, his death is what encouraged me to complete my weight loss.

Another benefit from using a fitness center is that many centers offer a service that has can determine your body mass index. Keeping track of your BMI is an excellent way to prevent weight regain. More effectively, it can show which percentages are from fat or muscle and track your progress.

Use a Personal Trainer

Joining a fitness center to lose weight and exercise publicly is not everyone's cup of tea. If you prefer to tackle your weight loss and activity regime on your own, consider hiring a personal trainer. The majority of personal trainers will work in private homes.

First, make sure that any personal trainer you want to hire has the educational and professional background needed to help you accomplish your goals. Because there is no standard licensing requirement for personal trainers, anyone can set up shop, including people who exercised in the past and decided that they had enough information to take on paying clients. Many colleges offer a curriculum in fields that prepare a professional personal trainer. These people know what exercises work and the reasons why, how to avoid injury, and what exercises are appropriate for different individuals.

A personal trainer who has not extensively interviewed you and shows up at your first session with a prepared but generic list of exercises is probably not going to be effective. You can get a list of exercises from the Internet, if that's all you want. What you are paying for is the trainer's expertise to ensure good results in your specific case and to avoid injury.

Work Out With a Friend

Everyone has friends who want to increase their activity level. Find someone suitable with similar goals and exercise together.

The amount of support you can receive increases with familiarity. People you know and care about are more likely to be helpful and honest than strangers. Your time together also provides an opportunity to get to know each other better, to share confidences, and to encourage each other to reach your activity goals.

Exercise and Support Groups

Bariatric support group meetings hold a room full of people who have been told to increase their activity level and who are highly motivated to do it. You can choose to work with someone who is about as far along their weight loss path as you are, or with someone who has achieved significant weight loss already and will help motivate you.

Be aware that people in support groups have a limited tolerance for anyone who does not make a sincere effort or who makes excuses for not achieving what is attempted. Their risk of failure increases if you fail, so don't expect saintly understanding and forgiveness if you aren't willing to make an effort. These people can also recognize an excuse for what it is – an avoidance mechanism – and a normal response to maintain their own motivation is to stop working with you and finding another partner instead.

People who are going through major life changes of their own can be very intolerant of anyone who sabotages their efforts, and rightfully so. If making a commitment and keeping it are problems for you, asking weight loss patients attending support groups to help you is probably a big mistake.

8

Support Groups

Bariatric surgeons agree that joining and participating in a bariatric support group is highly desirable in achieving long–term weight loss success.

While joining a support group is not compulsory, many bariatric teams view a reluctance to participating in support groups as an indicator that the patient is not serious about long term weight loss goals, or is viewing bariatric surgery as a "magic pill" that cures obesity with little or no effort.

Bariatric patients who join support groups have significant advantages over those who do not participate:

✓ Lap band patients who attended support groups achieved a 1.6 lower body mass index than those patients who did not.[1]

✓ Support group patients have a 10% lower BMI than non-support group patients.[2]

✓ Not only do support group attendees lose more weight, but the more often patients attend group meetings, the more weight they lose.

Support groups provide a resource to discuss problems or issues about weight loss surgery. The members of your support group are dealing with

1   Ehab Elakkary, Ali Elhorr, Faisal Aziz, M M Gazayerli and Yvan Silva. "Do Support Groups Play a Role in Weight Loss After Laparoscopic Adjustable Gastric Banding?" Obesity Surgery, March 2006. Vol 16, Num 3.

2   Whitney Orth, Atul Madan, Raymond Taddeucci, Mace Coday and David Tichansky. "Support Group Meeting Attendance is Associated With Better Weight Loss." Obesity Sur-

issues similar to the ones you'll face after surgery. They know what works and what does not work. They will hold you responsible for your actions in a compassionate and caring way.

The best reason for participating in a support group is that bariatric patients who self-monitor their progress are much less likely to regain weight following bariatric surgery.[3]

Bariatric support groups also help you maintain your motivation for losing weight and preventing weight regain.

The most effective support groups are those that you personally attend. Many bariatric surgeons participate with support groups, often hosting meetings and encouraging outside speakers. If you live in an area where a number of bariatric patients live, patients can form their own support group that is not affiliated with a particular bariatric surgeon. In most cases, patients who have had any type of weight loss surgery are encouraged to attend, even in groups hosted by specific bariatric surgeons.

It is often helpful to bring a family member or friend when you attend a support group meeting. They will have a better understanding of what to expect and methods for dealing with some of the many changes that will happen for you. If you live alone, a support group can become part of an extended circle of people who are, from the outset, understanding and encouraging.

Those who attend support groups get a visual impression of the weight loss progress, as well as stories of positive and negative aspects of the post-bariatric lifestyle. This post-surgery connection is so important that it is often suggested not to have weight loss surgery if your bariatric surgeon does not have a support group available, either through his own practice or an independent group located in the area. While online support groups can be helpful, it is difficult to duplicate the interpersonal connection that is found in attending a live meeting.

The first place to start looking for a bariatric support group is at your surgeon's office. Chances are good that your surgeon sponsors a group, especially since many bariatric surgeons use the support group as a marketing aid and also require prospective patients to attend a number of support group meetings before their surgery is scheduled. The hospital

gery, April 2008. Vol 18, Num 4.

3   J Odom, et al. "Behavioral Predictors of Weight Regain after Bariatric Surgery." Obesity Surgery, June 2009. DOI 10.1007/s11695-009-9895-6

or outpatient facility where your surgeon performs the surgery might sponsor a support group if enough people are interested in attending one. At the very least, the surgeon's office staff can refer you to outside groups with which they are not affiliated, since many support groups routinely make themselves known to bariatric surgeons in their area.

If your own bariatric surgeon cannot help with finding a group, consult other bariatric surgeons or nearby hospitals. Be wary of surgeons who do not acknowledge the benefit of attending support group meetings.

You can always start your own group if none exists in your geographical area. Your bariatric surgeon might be amenable to letting the group use his facility for meetings, or provide a staff member to act as moderator. In the support group I attended, my bariatric surgeon provided the meeting facilities (a large conference room space in a local hospital), brought in speakers, had staff members act as moderator and provided bottled water and samples of bariatric products like supplements and protein shakes.

Support groups can be in-person (usually the most effective over the long term) or virtual (online support groups). Additional support from family and friends is often also available.

Choosing a Support Group

To ensure compatibility with a prospective support group, keep these points in mind:

✓ Is the support group moderated by a bariatric professional? Moderators commonly include dieticians or nutritionists, bariatric nurses and mental health counselors.

✓ How big is the group? Larger groups tend to be more anonymous; smaller groups provide more attention and feedback to individuals than can be accomplished in a larger group.

✓ Is the support group specialized for specific types of bariatric surgery? If a group is focused on gastric band surgery and you had Roux-en-Y, the topics being discussed might not be a good fit for you. If your area has several support groups to choose from, start with the one specializing in the same type of surgery you had. In most areas, the groups are all-inclusive for different surgery types. Patients in these groups rely on other patients who have had similar surgeries and understand that some issues faced after other procedures might not apply to them.

✓ Do you feel welcome and comfortable attending the group meetings? Chances are that you will feel encouraged to discuss your problems only if you feel comfortable with other group members. If you don't, try to find another group.

✓ Is the group truly interested in hearing everyone's point of view, or is there an atmosphere where some viewpoints are acceptable but others are not? Everyone should be able to express himself without being criticized or chastised by the group. Opinions expressed in support groups do not have to be politically correct to be valid and respected by the group.

✓ Is participation encouraged? The most effective groups encourage everyone to participate. Every group risks being dominated by a small percentage of attendees. Effective moderators are good at encouraging shy or introverted people to join the discussions and in knowing how to sidetrack people who have more extensive needs.

✓ Are there guest speakers? Does the group bring in guest speakers who have experience in dealing with the topics being discussed? Or is it an open forum (moderated discussion) format?

✓ Is the group positive in tone? Support groups that turn into bitch-and-moan hand-wringing sessions rarely have a beneficial effect on those who attend. It's nice to be able to vent, but do you really want to sit through week after week listening to someone complain that they can't lose weight? It's counterproductive and it can encourage a defeatist attitude throughout the group. Again, an effective moderator will not enable this type of behavior.

Some groups use a buddy system, assigning two compatible people to work together when times get rough. Other groups have clothing swaps. Rapid weight loss means that you will soon be too thin for your current wardrobe, and as you continue to lose weight, buying new clothes constantly can be a financial drain. These groups recycle good quality clothing that participants have outgrown. Also, many support group members have useful contacts outside the group and can refer you to other people or groups if necessary. If you are happy with your group, you can include some of these features.

You can also use a virtual (online) support group.

✓ Participation should be free. There is no reason to pay fees to an online group; the fees are paid to the people who maintain the website, not to the participants who do almost all of the work.

✓ You can ask a question and receive answers or support when you need it, since online groups are available 24 hours a day, 7 days a week. With online support groups, you don't have to wait until next week's meeting to find an answer to a question.

✓ If there is no in-person support group near your home, an online group might be your only alternative.

✓ With online groups, you assume more responsibility for yourself. You will feel somewhat more isolated. It is important to maintain food diaries, personal journals, and so forth — things that are often second nature at in-person support group meetings.

Many people who attend an in-person support group also use online support groups and bariatric forums to supplement the in-person group. Online groups offer the benefit of people participating from far flung geographical areas, with vastly differing experiences.

Other Support Resources For Your New Lifestyle

WLS Lifestyles is a monthly magazine for people who have had weight loss surgery. It provides tools, tips, support and inspiration. It is available by subscription in print or online; the website offers free articles each month on various topics.

```
http://www.wlslifestyles.com
```

Bariatric TV is a website that features Toni Towe and Lynnda Shepherd, two weight loss surgery patients who have successfully maintained their respective 130- and 120-pound weight loss. They consider themselves "surgically altered freaks," but in a healthy way. (See the website for an explanation.) Their YouTube.com type broadcasts are funny, irreverent and informative. Bariatric TV offers great advice and the viewpoint of those who have fought the battle and won. It's highly recommended!

http://www.BariatricTV.com

9

Relationships and Bariatric Surgery

People are rarely surprised that their relationship with food changes after bariatric surgery.

What is surprising is that relationships with people also change. This can happen with any relationship – family, friends, coworkers, and significant others.

After bariatric surgery, the divorce rate is extremely high. Many people also change jobs.

Much of our lives involves food. We gather socially for family dinners, holidays and romantic dates — and all of these events are impacted by your altered dietary needs.

More surprising is how others change in the way they interact with you. As your body changes, you become more confident. People who never noticed you before begin to notice you. People you considered good friends can become jealous and critical. While some relationships grow stronger, others weaken and end.

Bariatric surgery often affects your romantic relationships more than others. Someone who has known you for a while has gotten used to seeing you in a certain light. For most bariatric patients, the period following their surgery is full of anxiety and doubt, which can cause you to act differently than before. The person that your partner thought you were is changing with every day, and humans are not particularly adept at handling emotional fear. If your relationship was a good one, it can become stronger; if it was not doing well or had unresolved issues, these changes can push you further apart.

In many cases, a spouse or significant other gets used to the overweight partner's appearance. When people lose weight and become more attractive, it can cause new feelings of jealousy and the sense that the formerly overweight partner now has options in relationships that were not available before. It is rare, however, for an overweight partner to have bariatric surgery just to increase the pool of prospective suitors. While most bariatric patients anticipate looking better than they did, finding a new relationship is not the driving force behind seeking the surgery and committing to all of the lifestyle changes needed to maintain the new look.

If your romantic relationship becomes increasingly difficult or hostile, consider getting relationship therapy with a psychologist or other mental health professional.

One of the problems associated with weight loss surgery is that while patients see the physical changes in the mirror every day, many of them still imagine themselves as being fat.

Some changes are beneficial. Many people who have been obese for a number of years have endured discrimination, felt helpless, and accepted situations that others would not have accepted or endured. Significant weight loss can help some of them learn to stand up for themselves and to expect to be treated better by those around them.

Coping With Relationship Changes

Here are some suggestions for coping with the changes in your relationships.

✓ Be mindful of the changes being experienced by the people around you. While they might have supported you in your quest for bariatric surgery, they are probably unsure of how to react to you as you change right in front of their eyes. Their world is changing too.

✓ Accept compliments gracefully, but do not focus on them. People who have not seen you in a while will easily notice the physical changes in your body. Those who are constantly around you might not notice the difference until it becomes more extreme. Allow people the space they need to adjust to the new you.

✓ Avoid talking about your weight loss surgery and subsequent success, since it can make you appear to be self-centered. Show enthusiasm for whatever is going on in the lives of your friends and family.

✓ As you lose weight, you will probably become more active and begin to try new activities. Include family and friends in the new interest.

✓ Compliment your significant other. Take the focus from you and your weight loss and ensure that others have their time to shine. Some people probably helped you to feel better at times before your surgery; return the favor.

✓ Do something special to make those around you feel special. Buy concert tickets or a CD, or plan a weekend vacation together. Don't wait for an occasion that necessitates gift-giving, like birthdays or holidays. Do it for no reason.

✓ Listen when friends and family want to discuss changes in you with which they are not comfortable. Don't take offense at what they say.

✓ Be empathic. Losing weight feels great, but the response from loved ones can be unpredictable.

Romantic Relationships and Bariatric Surgery

A study completed in 2008[1] found that weight loss surgery patients can encounter diverse relationship issues as they go through the bariatric process. Weight loss issues for couples can stem from the patients' and their partners' expectations, the patients' increase in energy, their enhanced confidence, and changes in appearance.

Changes in sexual intimacy, beliefs about the stability of the relationship and risk of divorce after weight loss surgery also remain common concerns.

Overall, the research suggests that weight loss surgery patients report improvements in relationship satisfaction and the quality of their sexual life after surgery, while experiencing minimal disruption to their marital relationships.

Suggestions were made for medical providers working with weight loss surgery patients on their relationship issues. These suggestions stress the need for communication, the importance of accurate information, recruiting support, and obtaining psychological counseling when needed.

Another study[2] noted that if both partners were of normal weight at the time they were married, they have a better chance of surviving the weight loss and associated disruptions. If either partner was significantly overweight when they married, the "new person" that results after the surgery is very different from the original, and that can cause problems.

Weight loss patients are more likely to leave an abusive relationship. The partner might begin to feel less comfortable as the formerly obese partner loses weight and becomes more attractive. The formerly obese partner might just decide that the relationship is not worth the effort and decide to leave it to find a better option.

From a medical standpoint, the usual determination of whether bariatric surgery is successful is if the patient loses 50% or more of excess body weight. But there is more to it than that. Someone who is significantly overweight can lose more than one hundred pounds but still be considerably overweight. While the bariatric surgeon will probably be pleased by the medical success, including resolution of some co-morbid

---

1   Katherine Applegate and Kelli Friedman. "The Impact of Weight Loss Surgery on Romantic Relationships." Bariatric Nursing and Surgical Patient Care. June 2008. Vol 3, Num 2.

2   Dan Orzech. "Counseling Bariatric Surgery Patients." Social Work Today, Vol 5, Num 6.

conditions, the surgery is not as successful psychologically: that person still feels (and acts) as if they are significantly overweight.

Since many people manage stress by feeding themselves, it is important to acknowledge this tendency and to learn alternative ways of expressing emotions like sadness or boredom.

Your social life also changes after bariatric surgery. Instead of meeting friends at restaurants and eating out, you will have to find other ways to maintain your friendships. You need to find places other than restaurants to congregate with your friends, and activities that do not involve food.

Some people let you know that they love you by feeding you (and especially by feeding you sweets). When your grandmother offers you a piece of the pie she knows you love, turning it down can insult her. How do you deal with these situations? Use honesty. Discuss your bariatric surgery with your grandmother so that she can find another way to express her affection for you. You must be willing to tell her that you cannot eat that food any longer. You must be willing to take special care to let the people around you know that you still care about them, but your diet is severely restricted now and it is just not possible to eat that particular food. Then stick to your guns!

Sex and the Bariatric Patient

Let's face it: after bariatric surgery, you don't automatically become a beauty queen or the town stud. But there are some correlations to seeing an improvement in your sex life as a side effect of weight loss surgery.

Obese men can suffer from erectile dysfunction. A clinical study published recently in the Journal of Sexual Medicine showed that obese men with erectile dysfunction had low levels of testosterone. As the severity of obesity increased, the testosterone levels further decreased. In addition, they often had higher levels of the female hormone estradiol.

Being overweight can also cause shortness of breath during sex or exercise, limiting duration or intensity.

Excess abdominal fat, cardiovascular disease, high blood lipids and type 2 diabetes all contribute to erectile dysfunction. The study linked sexual health in men with their physical health.

Women, on the other hand, report more sexual impairment than men, which can be related to low self-esteem, unsatisfactory relationships, social stigma or other psychological issues. Their sex drive is not as closely linked to hormones as in men.

The study noted that there is no correlation between having satisfactory sexual activity and being thin or overweight. There are many sexually active overweight people and many sexually inactive thin people.

Weight Loss Surgery and Body Image

Bariatric patients must make lifestyle and dietary changes; they must also change the way they perceive their own bodies. As pounds are shed, people begin responding to them in ways different than before their surgery. Romantic partners might expect more sex. Some patients have anxiety issues from the sudden attention being paid to them by strangers.

As the pounds disappear, a lot of excess skin is left behind. Some bariatric patients have body contouring surgery done by a plastic surgeon to remove the extra loose skin, but it is expensive and usually not covered by health insurance. The saggy, droopy image that stares back from the mirror can be a turn-off for the bariatric patient.

After many years of being overweight, it can take additional years before the person can look in a mirror and get an objective look at the revised image. Women, more than men, are impacted by body image. The drastic body changes encountered during the transition to a more normal weight can impact self-esteem and confidence.

After going through weight loss surgery, many patients initially worry about medical issues. As time passes, those worries lessen and they begin to see exactly how much excess hanging skin they are developing. Some people run to a plastic surgeon, while others seem to be just fine with their body changes and life goes on as before. Even those who have body contouring surgeries often dislike the body they see in the mirror; the procedures can cause extensive scars.

Weight Loss Surgery and Fertility

Women who are significantly obese can have problems with becoming pregnant or carrying a baby to term. Obese men can have reduced sperm counts. In either case, infertility can prove to be a major problem in a relationship.

If there is a chance that a woman might become pregnant soon after surgery, a restrictive surgery like adjustable gastric band surgery is usually preferred over a malabsorptive procedure. A woman should not attempt pregnancy for at least 18 months following Roux-en-Y or biliopancreatic diversion with duodenal switch surgeries because these maladaptive procedures will severely limit the nutrients available to the developing fetus. For the same reason, Roux-en-Y and biliopancreatic diversion with duodenal switch patients cannot rely on birth control pills, since the hormones they contain might not be correctly absorbed after surgery. Barrier contraceptives should be used instead.

Men should be aware that their potency can increase after massive weight loss.

10

Plastic Surgery

In 2007, before my bariatric surgery, I remember talking with a friend who had a biliopancreatic diversion with duodenal switch done a year earlier. She had gone to Brazil for the procedure, since at that time (2006) it was not being performed laparoscopically in the USA. A woman who had been through the same procedure about a year earlier was staying in the hospital at the same time. She was waiting for extensive plastic surgery (called a body lift) to remove excess skin left after losing 225 pounds. My friend showed me a photograph taken of the woman, lying on the floor, immersed in a gigantic puddle of excess skin that pooled around her in every direction. It was fascinating to think that someone actually had lost that much weight after undergoing the procedure I was contemplating, but also unsettling to see the results after such a success. I confess that it was not the pretty picture I held in my own mind about how one would look after successful bariatric surgery.

Weight loss surgery patients are told that they need to exercise. However, excess loose skin can interfere with their ability to exercise (or even move). The situation becomes a stalemate: you can't exercise because not enough weight was lost, and you can't lose enough weight because you cannot exercise. Bariatric surgery eliminates this problem, but introduces a new one: what seems like acres of excess skin that is unsightly, cumbersome, and generally in the way.

After a significant and relatively rapid weight loss, one potential unwanted side effect is excess skin. In most cases it is not a medical problem, but definitely can be an aesthetic one. After a year or more devoted to losing weight, you discover to your dismay that you still cannot wear revealing or form-fitting clothes.

When you gain ten or twenty pounds of extra weight, your skin stretches to accommodate this increase. When you lose this weight this skin, which is moderately elastic, can shrink enough to accommodate the weight loss.

However, after hundreds of pounds have stretched the skin over a number of years, as it does in many morbidly obese people, the excess skin stays much the same; it has grown to that size and it cannot contract enough to counterbalance the quantity of fat cells that were lost. When significant body weight is dropped rapidly, the skin does not have enough time to tighten. In cases where the weight loss is significant (more than one hundred pounds), excess skin is much more likely. People who lose 150 or 200 pounds (not uncommon with bariatric surgery) can have so much extra skin that it prevents normal movement. The weight of the excess skin can also cause spinal or other bone problems, back strain, and difficulty in walking. Surplus skin that hangs in folds and touches other skin areas can foster infection because it constantly stays moist. At the very least, excess skin on the arms, around the waist and in the thighs can prevent clothes from fitting well.

After being elated at successfully losing a hundred pounds or more, many weight loss patients still have a body that is not pleasing in shape and tone. Plastic surgery can resolve this issue, and its effects are long lasting if your weight loss is stable at your goal weight. (Expect slight changes as the body naturally becomes less firm with age.)

I remember after losing a significant amount of weight in the late 1980s, my mother, a woman who was never afraid to share her opinion, remarked that my skin resembled the draperies at Torsone's, the local funeral parlor. Loose crepe-like skin is normal after massive weight loss. The only place on the planet where this does not seem to apply is Hollywood, where everyone seems to stay science-fiction young forever — another testament to the incredible power of plastic surgery!

Each person's skin reacts differently. Some people lose an astonishing amount of weight and their skin seems to fit well on their new body, while other people lose fewer pounds and end up looking like a shar-pei dog. Genetics plays a part in this scenario, as does age, environment, general health, how far the skin was stretched and how quickly the excess weight was gained. Faster weight gain results in stretched skin; if you already have stretch marks on your body, your skin is less elastic and will not shrink sufficiently. Stretch marks are actually a form of scar formed when tears in the skin caused by stretching heal together. Like any scar, they are permanent.

The skin's natural ability to stretch is a benefit — it prevents us from having to shed our skin as we grow from infant to adult. Its ability to contract naturally is useful, such as after childbirth. Skin is like a rubber band. When you gain weight, it's like pulling on a rubber band: it stretches to accommodate the increase. However, if you leave a rubber band on a large package for a length of time and then remove it, the band will often be flaccid and not contract back to its original size.

In general, bariatric patients focus on getting back to a normal size; very few anticipate the disappointment they will feel when their stretched skin fails to snap back into place.

As we age, our skin naturally becomes less elastic. Older bariatric patients can expect more excess skin. Younger patients with more than 100 pound losses can also expect to have excess skin.

Those who are bigger before their weight loss will develop more loose skin than those who have less to lose.

Different bariatric plastic surgery procedures are used for android and gynoid obesity profiles. Bodies store weight primarily in two different ways. *Android obesity* is displayed in a body profile that resembles an apple — the midsection is rounded evenly, or the stomach protrudes considerably. *Gynoid obesity* is displayed in a body profile that resembles a pear – the upper torso is smaller and the lower abdomen and hips carry most of the excess weight. While both sexes can have either profile, men tend towards android obesity and women tend to be gynoid obese.

After massive weight loss, body contouring plastic surgery can remove some of the excess fat and skin from the areas where it is associated with each type of obesity profile, creating a new body profile that is more evenly distributed and pleasingly contoured.

Your genetics also play a part in determining whether you have loose skin after your weight loss. Some people are predisposed to having loose skin or developing stretch marks that indicate skin that will not easily snap back into place. If your parents or grandparents had significant skin wrinkling, it might be genetically connected.

For weight loss surgery patients, even minor amounts of sagging skin folds can stay moist and harbor bacteria, leading to chronic skin infections that are impossible to treat without reconstructive plastic surgery.

For some patients, the need to have their excess skin removed is primarily a psychological one. Some patients feel fat even though they have lost a massive amount of weight and had excellent skin elasticity. And some patients need to have the last vestiges of their obesity removed in order to feel satisfaction and completion of the weight loss process. These people intend for the weight loss to be a permanent change.

Simple liposuction is not an option for the majority of weight loss patients. Liposuction removes fat deposits, but does nothing for skin that is stretched. In fact, having only liposuction can make the excess skin look worse because it removes some of the underlying structure.

While plastic surgery procedures for weight loss patients create scars (often very long ones), the scars are often hidden along natural folds in the body or in areas normally covered by clothing or underwear. Notable exceptions are arm and inner thigh lift scars, which extend down the inside of the arm or inside of the leg, but even these scars become quite unnoticeable after a couple of years. With plastic surgery, you trade "skin for scars." For those who have had massive weight loss and have large amounts of loose, droopy skin, this exchange is probably a happy one.

Whether you need plastic surgery to correct physical problems and medical conditions or to satisfy an emotional need, weight loss patients who have plastic surgery are, as a group, highly satisfied with their outcomes.

When To Have Plastic Surgery

Plastic surgeons advise people to wait for at least one year after weight loss surgery before having plastic surgery. Most plastic surgeons plan the surgery for no sooner than 18 months after your bariatric procedure. This is important for several reasons. Co-morbid conditions can improve in the year following weight loss surgery, reducing your risk for any type of surgery. Nutritional deficiencies can cause problems; patients have proven to be more compliant with nutritional guidelines if they plan to have plastic surgery. Also, your skin can shrink slightly as you maintain a lowered weight, which means less excess skin must be removed during the plastic surgery. It can also take a year to balance yourself out emotionally and psychologically so that you are ready for the physical changes that plastic surgery causes.

Other indicators can include waiting until:

✓ After you have reached your goal weight (or, for some plastic surgeons, lost at least 50% of your excess weight) and have maintained that weight for a year to 18 months.

✓ Your BMI is between 17 and 25 and has stabilized there for several months. You must be committed to maintaining that BMI.

✓ Your co-morbid conditions must be controlled or eliminated by the time you have plastic surgery. This reduces the chance of complications and minimizes any additional risks. Co-morbidities also increase the risk of problems with anesthesia.

Women who plan to have children are advised to postpone their plastic surgery until after childbearing. Pregnancy often causes weight gain and can negate some of the benefits of an abdominoplasty.

Before surgery, you should continue to eat in a healthy way and participate in an exercise program. After surgery, your exercise will be restricted to walking for the first four to six weeks, after which mild to moderate exercise can be resumed.

You will not be allowed to lift more than five or ten pounds for several weeks.

If you smoke, you must stop smoking for at least a month prior to surgery. Smokers have much higher risks from complications of anesthesia, blood clotting, and other issues. The healing times required for smokers is also longer than with non-smokers. Avoid second-hand smoke during this period and for several weeks after your surgery. You must also stop all recreational drug usage and refrain from consuming alcohol, since both interfere with blood clotting. If you use anabolic steroids, completely discontinue using them a minimum of six weeks before surgery.

You must also be advised about medications that need to be changed, discontinued, or have the dosage adjusted. Certain medications, such as blood-thinners, aspirin and non-steroidal anti-inflammatory drugs (NSAIDs) must be discontinued. Certain vitamins and homeopathic remedies must also be stopped, since they too can interfere with normal blood clotting times or promote bleeding. You might also have to change the dosage or stop taking other prescription medications; this should be discussed with your plastic surgeon and prescribing physician before making the medication changes.

Choosing a Plastic Surgeon

There is a difference between plastic surgeons who primarily do cosmetic enhancement procedures like collagen lips or eyelid lifts and the plastic surgeons who perform full body lifts. Look for a surgeon who has had instruction and education in post-bariatric body contouring and body lift procedures provided by organizations such as the American Society of Plastic Surgeons and the American Society for Aesthetic Plastic Surgery. While there are more than 150 self-designated boards, only a handful are designated by the American Board of Medical Specialties (ABMS), such as the American Board of Plastic Surgery.

Here are some tips to consider when choosing a plastic surgeon:

✓ Review the doctor's qualifications, including education and training, the type and origin of certification held, and the number of similar procedures performed.

✓ View before and after pictures of patients who have undergone the type of surgery you contemplate. Ask to speak to some of these patients about their experiences.

✓ Ask the surgeon what is planned in your specific case (not how similar procedures are generally done).

✓ Discuss any possible complications and understand the level of risk for each of them.

✓ Ask where the procedure will be performed. It should be done in an accredited facility. Is it an outpatient facility, or will you be admitted to a hospital?

✓ Ask about the type of anesthesia that is used, and about how long it will take.

✓ Ask about pre-surgical and post-surgical instructions.

✓ Ask about any medication changes that must be made before and after surgery.

✓ Ask about the surgeon's policy if the procedure needs to be repeated or when a secondary procedure is required.

Preventing Excess Skin

To prevent excess skin, follow these suggestions:

✓ **Lose weight gradually.** Although most people want their weight loss to be as rapid as possible, losing it more slowly gives the body the time it needs to gradually tighten the skin as the fat cells shrink. A weight loss of one to two pounds per week is optimal. If you lose 5 pounds a week, you will lose 80 pounds in 4 months, which will result in loose hanging skin. Also, losing weight more gradually often translates into better long-term success.

✓ **Buy a good quality commercial skin tightening cream and use it.** Look for products that contain vitamin C and copper. Buy the best quality cream that you can afford. Apply the cream regularly according to package directions. Note that some skin tightening creams can irritate the skin; try a different brand if this happens.

✓ **Exercise.** As you lose fat cells, you will add and tone the muscle cells. People who are overweight usually do not exercise enough. Weight loss combined with poor muscle tone creates an emaciated look that emphasizes excess skin (sometimes called the "prisoner of war effect").

Preventing Skin Surgery

✓ **Increase your exercise level and include muscle toning and strengthening.** Building muscle tone keeps skin firmer and tighter. Include exercises such as weight lifting and resistance training to increase muscle size and tone; add stamina-building exercise like Pilates or yoga to increase tone and stamina.

✓ **Remember that some bariatric surgical procedures involve malabsorption of nutrients.** If you had this type of surgery, it is essential that you increase your intake of vitamins, minerals and essential fatty acids. You will probably be instructed to use supplements to maintain necessary levels of these nutrients. You can also add fish, fruits, vegetables, nuts and complex carbohydrates to your diet to get more nutrients from natural sources.

✓ **Post-bariatric patients can become dehydrated.** Dehydrated skin is more likely to hang loosely than hydrated skin. Drink 6 to 8 glasses of water a day to stay hydrated.

✓ **Eat 4 to 8 small meals a day.** This is necessary because the smaller stomach pouch cannot hold enough food at one time for your needs. Your smaller stomach pouch makes it difficult to get enough nutrition if you eat only 3 meals a day. Remember that the additional meals are going to be meals, not high calorie snacks. You will simply divide the portions of a regular meal and eat them at different times.

Removing Excess Skin

Besides the aesthetic issue of loose excess skin being unsightly, it can hinder movement or cause discomfort. Skin that rubs or chafes can cause medical problems. For many, removing excess skin can be the final step in the weight loss process. This is done with plastic surgery and can range from inexpensive simple procedures to costly full body lifts.

If you decide to investigate the possibility of having your excess skin removed, consider these points:

✓ **Determine how you will pay for the plastic surgery.** It is generally not covered by health insurance unless the excess skin is causing a medical problem that cannot be improved through other methods. Some health insurance plans cover this type of surgery (see "Health Insurance and Excess Skin" on page 98).

✓ **Choose a plastic surgeon who routinely performs full body lifts if you need extensive work done.** Plastic surgeons often specialize in specific procedures. A body lift is a series of procedures (that can be combined into a single procedure in some cases) to remove excess skin from several locations on the body after bariatric surgery. It is a long and complicated surgery with significant risk. Movement after surgery is severely restricted for a long period of time because the body heals slowly after such extensive work; you will not be going back to work within a few days of this type of surgery.

✓ **Ask your bariatric surgeon for a referral to a plastic surgeon.** Many bariatric surgeons have cooperative affiliations with plastic surgeons because so many patients opt for plastic surgery after their weight loss.

✓ **Choosing a plastic surgeon just because he offers bargain prices is inadvisable.** The work done by plastic surgeons is visible; this is not the place to cut corners or try to save a few dollars. Plastic surgery can have severe complications, so you need to choose from among the very best surgeons. If you can't afford the best, put the surgery on hold temporarily while you continue to save money to pay for it.

✓ **Consult with a plastic surgeon to discuss what can be done.** The surgeon will also discuss any limitations to this type of surgery.

✓ **Discuss with the plastic surgeon the types of surgery you are contemplating.** These can include tummy tucks, buttocks lifts, thigh lifts, and arm lifts. Women often have breast lifts and implants.

✓ **Determine how many procedures you will have.** Full body lifts can be done in a series of separate procedures (staged reconstruction). This is often recommended for patients with health issues, which includes a large number of bariatric patients, since many had the bariatric surgery in order to ameliorate other health issues. Danger or complications from anesthesia increases as the length of a surgical procedure increases, especially after 4 to 6 hours of anesthesia.

Anesthesia risks usually require patients having full body lifts to be admitted to a hospital, where other surgical specialists are available immediately if a problem arises, since risk is significantly increased for longer surgeries like full body lifts.

Co-morbid conditions, including hypertension, coronary disease, diabetes, sleep apnea, venous insufficiency and malnutrition, can remain problematical even after weight loss. Your plastic surgeon can require you to consult with specialists for medical clearance before surgery and to be carefully monitored after surgery.

Many plastic surgeons advise staged reconstruction surgeries instead of full body lifts for weight loss patients, in which several surgeries are done sequentially. This process reduces the amount of time spent under anesthesia and reduces other surgical risks that can be caused by complications of co–morbid conditions. The recovery period after a staged procedure is less than after a full body lift, simply because it is difficult for the body to heal several lengthy incisions all at the same time.

Some procedures should be done in a specific order before or after other procedures. For example, if you plan to have a breast enhancement, body lift and thigh lift, the body lift should be done first, since it also helps lift the thighs. The skin on the abdomen is tightened, which pulls downward on the breasts and changes the contour of the torso. If the breast lift was done first, the new breasts could end up further down the chest than they should, requiring a revisional breast lift to put them back where they should be.

Body lifts require a minimum of several weeks away from work. Some require one or more months of recuperation. Single procedures usually heal more quickly than full body lifts. and have shorter recovery periods.

Plastic surgery on the body, including full body lifts, is painful. While pain can be managed effectively with medication, full body lifts are among the most painful of plastic surgeries.

Arrange for nursing care after your surgery. This can be a professional nurse, a family member or just a friend, depending on how extensive your surgery will be. For the first few days or weeks after your surgery, you will be restricted in activity level and intensity.

Many of the procedures require drainage tubes to be inserted into the incision, which often stay in place for about two weeks and require care at home. They are removed when the volume of drainage is low.

You might have to wear a medical compression garment at all times except while showering. This should be worn until your surgeon tells you it is no longer necessary.

Dressings are usually removed about two days after surgery, after which you can begin showering.

You must take the same care and diligence in finding an excellent plastic surgeon as you did to find your bariatric surgeon.

You must also have realistic expectations about the cosmetic surgery. This type of surgery can improve your appearance after you lose weight, but like weight loss surgery, it is not a miracle cure. The cost of high quality plastic surgery can make it necessary to have fewer or less complicated procedures than you might like.

Health Insurance and Excess Skin

Very few health insurance plans will pay for plastic surgery that is performed for aesthetic improvement. Many plans, however, cover certain plastic surgical procedures commonly performed on post-bariatric patients if the surgery is medically necessary.

If you need to have loose excess skin removed because it is causing medical problems, like chafing, infection, or back discomfort, health insurance plans (including Medicare and Medicaid) will consider paying for the surgery.

It is important to choose both bariatric and plastic surgeons who accept your health insurance plan. It is also important to choose a surgeon who knows what must be submitted to the insurance company in order to obtain the necessary approvals.

Many health insurance plans routinely deny coverage for any plastic surgery. The denials are based on the surgery being performed only for cosmetic reasons; other types of cosmetic improvements, such as tooth veneers, are not covered by insurance. Read the coverage data that your plan sent you as part of your contract with them; if there is a possibility that the surgery you seek can be covered, ask your surgeons (both bariatric and plastic) to submit the information to the plan that proves medical necessity, and be prepared to appeal a routine denial if necessary.

Health insurance plans cover only the types of plastic surgery that are medically necessary in your case. If you have any aesthetic work done at the same time, costs for that part of the surgery will not be covered. In some cases, health plans are generous; for example, some plans allow either an abdominoplasty or a panniculectomy, while others will reimburse only for certain types of surgeries, only for specific reasons, and will not offer alternatives. Each plan is different, so check with your health insurance company before committing to any surgery to see exactly what is covered and under which circumstances reimbursement might be possible. Your surgeon's office is familiar with dealing with insurance plans and can help you with this task.

Medicare

Medicare is a health insurance program that is administered by the federal government's Social Security division. Like other health insurance plans, many of the same guidelines apply, although coverage amounts can vary from the levels provided by private insurance plans.

Medicare covers both bariatric surgery and post-bariatric medically necessary plastic surgery as long as their guidelines are observed. If you have Medicare, you can request a predetermination of benefit eligibility before beginning the bariatric process.

Medicaid and State-level Health Insurance

Medicaid is a state-level health insurance program. Several other health insurance programs exist and can vary from state to state. Since each state controls its own programs, including eligibility guidelines and coverage, you must contact the appropriate agency in your state to determine if any of the programs can be useful to you.

In many states, Medicaid coverage is similar to that provided through the federal Medicare program, so bariatric and plastic surgeries might be covered in your state if they are medically necessary. Applying for these benefits and receiving approval can take a significant amount of time, which must be factored into your plans. Coverage for the same procedure varies by state, and often within different counties in a state, depending on how the programs are funded.

Body Contouring Surgical Procedures

Body contouring surgery, as the term is used here, refers to a series of surgical procedures that eliminate or reduce excess skin and fat that remains after obese people lose a significant amount of weight in a variety of locations on the body, including the torso, upper arms, chest and thighs.

Body contouring surgery consists of a number of plastic surgery procedures, including arm lifts, thigh lifts, abdominoplasty or panniculectomy, back lifts, and various enhancement surgeries.

Abdominoplasty

An abdominoplasty is often called a "tummy tuck." In this procedure, loose abdominal muscles are tightened and excess abdominal skin is removed. Liposuction can be used to remove excess fat cells from the abdomen. This surgery is the most popular procedure performed after massive weight loss because the end results are dramatic. This surgery can improve the shape and contour of the abdomen when weight loss and exercise are not enough.

An incision is made that extends from hipbone to hipbone around the waist. The surgeon removes any excess fat, either excising it directly or using liposuction, and then stitches the abdominal muscles together to tighten them. The navel is repositioned to an appropriate place, and the excess skin is removed. In some cases, a second vertical incision is made to remove excess skin from the upper abdomen. Drainage tubes are inserted and the incision is closed.

The procedure for a panniculectomy is very similar (except for tightening the abdominal muscles, which is not done in panniculectomies). For more information, see "Panniculectomy" on page 112.

Arm Lift (Brachioplasty)

The extra flesh on the arms of bariatric patients almost always appears on the underside of the upper arm and is sometimes referred to as "bat wings." This excess skin can prevent sleeved garments from fitting properly and cause underarm skin rash and irritation. The skin on the inner area of the upper arm is tender and stretches easily, often leaving stretch marks and excess droopy skin that does not conform to a slimmer upper arm.

This surgery is not advised for people who have *Hidradenitis Suppurativa*, a persistent infection of the sweat glands in the armpit, or for women who have had radical mastectomies or extensive breast cancer, since they are at risk of developing chronic arm swelling after this surgery.

Surgeons make decisions on the underside of the arm from the armpits to the elbow to remove the excess skin. Some surgeons extend the incision into the armpit and onto the upper chest. The incision can be on the inner part of the arm, which is usually held close to the body, or on the bottom. The resulting scar is fairly well hidden and can be covered with clothing.

As with any plastic surgery, arm lift patients should expect restrictions on lifting weights over 5 pounds, issues with swelling and bruising, and pain. Pain lasts from 7 to 10 days after surgery and is treated with pain medication. Your hands might tingle slightly, and use of the hands is severely limited; you might have problems trying to do simple tasks like tying shoes, fastening buttons or writing. Recovery time requires several weeks, during which the movement of the arms is restricted. Stitches are removed a few days after surgery, and showering is possible a day or two after surgery. Your arms will feel uncomfortable and tight after surgery, but this sensation disappears after a few days. Compression garments are usually worn for a short period to reduce swelling and promote healing. Some surgeons prefer their patients to keep their arms held in an elevated position (above the heart) for several days to reduce swelling and the chance of developing blood clots. During this time, your ability to perform normal everyday tasks is severely limited.

Augmentation Surgery

Several surgical procedures are used to improve the appearance of parts of the body after massive weight loss, including:

Bicep and Tricep Augmentation

Soft solid silicone implants are used to augment the biceps and triceps muscles in the upper arm, providing increased mass and adding muscular definition.

For augmentation surgery, a 1 to 2 inch incision is made in the upper arm near the armpit. The silicone implant is placed and the incision is closed. The surgery lasts about two hours and can be done under local anesthesia in an outpatient facility or general anesthesia in a hospital. Stitches are usually removed about two days after surgery. You can expect issues with pain, swelling and bruising, as with any plastic surgery. Moving the arms is difficult during the first week following surgery. While the scar heals in about ten days, the tissues in the arm take about six to ten weeks to recuperate. It is essential to follow the surgeon's advice regarding activity and exercise levels during this period. Implants are relatively stable after they have healed in place, but can be displaced or damaged if an injury occurs of the type that would cause muscle injury or bone breakage.

These procedures can be done as a part of an arm lift to improve the contour and definition of the upper arm. The longer incision on the inside or bottom of the upper arm can be used to insert the implants.

Buttocks Lift and Buttocks Enhancement

A buttocks lift is used to remove excess fat and skin from the buttocks, improving the contour of the waist, hips and back of the thighs. Excess fat and skin is trimmed away from the thighs and the buttocks which leaves a more toned and flatter looking rear. The incision for this surgery is across the lower back, from hip to hip. The surgeon pulls the excess skin below the incision to lift the buttocks and outer thighs. The excess skin is removed. The surgery takes about two hours under general anesthesia. Abdominal compression garments or binders are worn for about six weeks to avoid swelling and to support the area during healing. Swelling can last for up to three months. There can be mild to moderate postoperative pain that is controlled by medication.

Some post-weight loss patients feel that their buttocks are too flat and opt for buttock augmentation, using solid silicone implants or with body fat removed from other areas of the body. The surgery is performed under general anesthesia, usually in an outpatient facility and takes 2 to 3 hours to complete.

For buttocks enhancement surgery, the incision for the implants is made between the buttocks and the resulting scar is hidden by the natural contours of the body.

The implants round out the upper and outer portions of the buttocks. To reshape the lower portion, fat injections are used. This procedure is done at another time from the silicone implants to avoid the possibility of the injected fat causing infections and because the pressure of the implants can destroy the fat.

The surgery can be painful, with swelling that often requires drainage. Sitting will be uncomfortable for a period of time.

Calf Implants

Some people are not happy with the way their calves appear, especially if their calves are thin or shapeless. People who have had massive weight loss and who carried significant weight in their lower legs often opt for this procedure after having the excess skin removed.

Soft silicone implants can be placed to improve the muscular definition of the calf area. These implants are also used to make the calves more symmetrical. It is usually performed under local anesthesia, but can also be done with general anesthesia. Small incisions are made behind the knee and the implants are placed. The scar is usually small and hidden behind the bend of the knee. Recovery, however, can be painful and lengthy, taking several weeks. Walking is extremely difficult at first; walking with flat shoes or with no shoes can be quite painful for several weeks. Women are often advised to wear high heels during the recovery period to reduce swelling, and the legs should be elevated for the same reason. Compression stockings or ace bandages can help to reduce swelling. Avoid exercise for several weeks and running for up to three months.

Pectoral Implants

Many men find that after massive weight loss, some muscle mass in the chest is also lost. Even after increasing the amount of exercise, a chest can be flatter or less bulky than desired. Solid silicone pectoral implants can be used to increase the bulk of the chest and mimic well-developed pectoral muscles. Pectoral implants provide additional bulk but do not improve muscle definition.

An incision is made, usually in the armpit, and a pocket is created in the pectoral muscle. The silicone implant is sculpted to fit the patient, inserted under a layer of muscle and sewn in place. The incision is closed and covered with a small dressing to promote healing.

After the surgery, arm movement is restricted to avoid shifting the implants. Expect some pain and minor swelling, which can be controlled with medication.

Health insurance plans pay for pectoral implants to correct congenital deformity or to repair an injury, but usually do not cover the surgery when it is done to improve appearance after weight loss.

Back Lift

Back lifts are used to smooth sagging skin on the back and sides of the body. Liposuction can be used to remove underlying pockets of fat.

An incision is made at the bottom of the back, usually under the underwear line below the waist. The excess skin on the back is stretched downwards, excess skin is removed and the incision is closed.

This surgery can be performed on men, who tend not to develop as much sagging skin on the back as women.

Bra Line Back Lift

A newer form of back lift is called a bra line back lift. In this surgery, an incision is made across the back at breast height. At some point before surgery, you will be asked to wear a bra or swimsuit top so that the surgeon can mark the appropriate incision line to ensure that it will be covered by clothing.

If this surgery is performed correctly and the patient follows the surgeon's advice for post-surgical wound care, the fine high quality scar that results is hidden under the bra line.

General anesthesia is used. You will be admitted to a hospital or an outpatient facility, depending on your medical history and needs. The surgery takes about one hour.

The surgery has a short recovery time and low complication rates, along with a scar that can be easily hidden or is marginally noticeable. While it can be done on men, the scar is much more visible than that from a back lift, since on men it cannot be hidden beneath a bra or halter top. For this reason, it is rarely performed on men.

You can wear a bra or other garment after the first week. Choose a comfortable bra with a wide transverse strap to avoid putting too much pressure on the incision.

Avoid vigorous exercise, lifting items heavier than 5 or 10 pounds, flexing or stretching the back, bending at the waist and raising your arms over your head. You can begin showering the day after surgery (follow your surgeon's advice) and must avoid submerging the incision in water — no bathing, swimming or soaking in a jacuzzi.

Breast Lift and Breast Implants

A breast lift counteracts sagging breasts and restores them to a more natural shape. Some women opt for breast implants, which add volume and fullness to the breasts.

Women naturally store extra fat in the breasts. Women who have been morbidly obese and then lost a significant amount of weight find that much of the lost fat was in the breasts, which now sag and droop down onto the upper abdomen.

Plastic surgeons define breast sagging (ptosis) using the position of the nipples on the breast mount. Women whose nipples are at the breast mount have mild ptosis. Women whose nipples droop below the level of the breast crease have moderate ptosis. In advanced ptosis, the nipples have dropped below the level of the breast mount and are at the level of maximum breast projection. In severe ptosis, the nipples have dropped below the breast mount and are pointing at the floor.

Surgery removes excess skin and moves the nipples to a higher position on the chest. Different procedures are used, depending on the severity of the breast ptosis. For mild ptosis, during a crescent lift, the surgeon removes an area of crescent-shaped skin above the areola and raises the remaining breast skin to a higher position. For moderate ptosis, using a concentric lift, the surgeon makes two circular incisions around the areola, then removes the donut-shaped excess skin and stitches the surrounding skin to the areola. Neither of these techniques works well for women who have had massive weight loss and have significant excess skin on the breast.

The anchor-shaped mastopexy is the most common procedure, as well as being the most invasive. The surgeon makes an incision shaped like a boat anchor with a circle at the top. The nipple is placed in the circle at the top of the anchor, creating the shape of the new breast. The lines at the bottom form the lower contour of the new breast. The surgeon pulls the skin sections together and stitches them closed.

Breast lifts can be done in conjunction with breast augmentation, during which soft silicone implants are inserted into the breast to increase volume and fullness. Implants can be used to improve the contours of the breast. It can also be combined with breast reduction surgery to reduce the overall size of the breasts while improving their appearance.

While women who have not been overweight can have a mini breast lift, where only the nipple is repositioned, this surgery is not extensive enough to correct the excess hanging breast skin seen on women who have lost massive amounts of weight.

After breast lift surgery, you will wear a compression garment for a minimum of several weeks. This reduces swelling and ensures that the new breasts heal in the proper place. Using some form of bra or other garment which provides support to the breast tissue is recommended for the year following surgery; your surgeon might suggest that you continue wearing this type of garment permanently for the best results.

If you plan to have a body lift, have the breast lift after the body lift is complete and healed. This ensures that your new breasts will remain in the correct position after all of your surgeries are completed.

As with any plastic surgery, you can expect some pain, swelling and bruising. Your activities will be restricted, along with lifting restrictions of more than 5 pounds. Exercise is limited for a few weeks. Your breasts might feel tight or uncomfortable at first; this sensation disappears with time. You must keep any dressings dry and change them according to the surgeon's orders. If drains were inserted, you will clean them at home; they are removed a few days or a week after surgery, depending on how well you are healing. You can resume showering about two or three days after surgery but avoid bathing, swimming or soaking in a jacuzzi.

Breast lifts and breast reductions are sometimes covered by health insurance plans if there is an associated medical reason for the surgery. Breast enhancement surgery is not covered since it is elective cosmetic surgery. You can ask your surgeon's office to help you with reimbursement issues before surgery, since they are aware of the requirements of many insurance plans.

Face Lift

If your face was very full or round before your weight loss, you might be left with loose flesh on the cheeks or drooping jowls. A face lift procedure can remove the excess skin and fat deposits.

Few bariatric patients are reimbursed for any form of facial plastic surgery after weight loss since it is an elective cosmetic procedure. It is also very difficult to attempt to justify medical issues associated with weight loss that would require this type of plastic surgery. You should expect to pay for a face lift yourself, or use a financing plan offered by most plastic surgeons.

It is not unusual for weight loss patients who have lost massive amounts of weight and then had one or more plastic surgery procedures to reconstruct their body to get through that process and discover that they are still unhappy with the face looking back at them in the mirror.

Face lifts for weight loss patients often include neck lifts, since the neck and throat often have sagging loose skin or "turkey wattles" after massive weight loss. In some cases, having a neck lift instead of a face lift might produce better results. For more information, see "Neck Lift (Platysmaplasty)" on page 112.

New methods for doing face lifts are easier to perform, less invasive, and can be done as an outpatient, making a face lift much less expensive than in the past.

Liposuction

This is one of the most popular cosmetic surgery options. A cannula is inserted through small incisions into the area where fat is to be removed. The cannula breaks up the fat deposits using a series of push and pull movements. A vacuum pump or syringe attached to the other end of the cannula removes the broken-down fat cells.

Liposuction is often performed on the abdomen, hips, thighs, buttocks or arms for weight loss patients in conjunction with other more extensive procedures. Having liposuction alone will not resolve sagging excess skin issues and can actually worsen the area's appearance. Liposuction is designed to remove excess fat; it is normal to have a small amount fat in the body of even those who are very physically fit.

Lower Body Lift

When people gain a lot of weight, they often store it around their entire body, which includes the front, sides and back, in the area between the bottom of the ribs to the pelvic region. When weight is lost, a considerable amount of excess fat and skin is left in this region. While it is most obvious from the front, it also extends around both sides and onto the lower back and upper buttocks. This type of excess skin and fat is called *circumferential excess*.

To treat circumferential excess in patients with massive weight loss, a *belt lipectomy* or *lower body lift* is performed. In this procedure, a wedge of tissue that goes around the body at the hips is removed.

While an abdominoplasty (tummy tuck) treats only the front of the body, a belt lipectomy addresses the issue of the excess fat and skin on the hips and back. In the front, the excess fat and skin is removed and often the underlying muscles of the abdominal wall are tightened. The patient is turned over on the operating table so that the surgical team can work on the sides and back of the body. Liposuction can be done on the thighs or upper abdomen to reduce their size and flatten them further. The scar that results is thong-shaped for most surgeons, following just inside the waistband and leg openings of the underwear so that the entire scar usually can be hidden by minimal clothing or a bathing suit. In some cases, the incision must be placed where the scar is more visible.

In this surgery:

✓ the hanging apron of extra fat and skin on the stomach (the *pannicula*) is eliminated

✓ the abdomen is flattened, although to a greater degree if the abdominal muscles are tightened

✓ the drooping pubic region is pulled up and flattened

✓ a waist is created

✓ the thighs are lifted and contoured

✓ the buttocks are lifted and contoured

Recovery from a lower body lift takes 3 to 4 weeks. Many surgeons prefer to use compression garments after the surgery to reduce swelling and ensure that everything stays in place until it heals. The incision is a long one, extending almost all the way around the body, and patients are advised to walk bent at the waist for a week or so to avoid putting too much tension on the stitches. This surgery frequently requires the placement of drainage tubes, which must be monitored, cleaned regularly and kept sterile. They are left in place for a few days to a few weeks, depending on the patient. While you will see a big improvement almost immediately after surgery, the final effects of the surgery will not occur until about a year after the surgery, when the body has completely healed and the tendency to swell has stopped.

You will be advised to take pain medication for a short period after surgery, ranging from several days to several weeks, although pain resolves with healing and a reduction in swelling. This is an extensive surgery, requiring several hours under anesthesia and involving a large portion of the body; recovery takes several weeks. Activity and exercise must be severely curtailed during this period. Lower body lifts are almost always performed in hospitals with general anesthesia and require a short hospital stay.

Male Breast Reduction (Gynecomastia)

Some men find that they are left with what looks like sagging breasts after losing a great deal of weight. They often are left with stubborn areas of fat in the chest area which resemble female breasts, a condition called *gynecomastia*.

Fat cells, especially when present in large numbers, convert the male hormone testosterone into the female hormone estrogen, which stimulates breast growth. Testosterone deficiencies that develop normally with age can also contribute to gynecomastia. This condition is seen in males of all ages, and it can either resolve itself as time passes or need surgical correction.

However, in men who have massive weight loss, the problem is usually excess fat cells that are resistant to efforts made in the diet. Unfortunately, exercise does not help either type.

With massive weight gain, some residual fat cells can remain in the breast or nipple area and can be removed only with surgery. Breasts that are enlarged due to fat deposits actually have a condition called *pseudogynecomastia*.

Note: gynecomastia results in breasts that are enlarged, but both are the same size and flabby. If the problem exists only in one breast and it is firm or hard, it can be male breast cancer. This condition is often hidden by massive excess weight; when weight is lost, the condition is easier to reveal and diagnose. You should see a surgeon immediately if you have these symptoms.

For the surgery to be effective, you must be at a stable goal weight for a year. Many drugs can cause gynecomastia; if you use any of these drugs, you will make a poor candidate for this surgery:

✓ anti-androgens used to treat prostate enlargement or cancer and some other conditions

✓ AIDS medications

✓ anti-anxiety medications

✓ tricyclic antidepressants

✓ antibiotics

✓ ulcer medications

✓ cancer treatments

✓ heart medications

✓ anabolic steroids and androgens

✓ alcohol

✓ amphetamines

✓ marijuana

✓ heroin

In this procedure, an incision is made around the outside edge of the areola. Excess breast tissue is removed with a scalpel. If only fat needs to be removed, small stab incisions are used to remove fat deposits with liposuction. This small incision, usually less than half an inch, is made in the edge of the areola. Some surgeons prefer to make the incision in the armpit, which is slightly less visible. You might feel a vibration or friction during the procedure, but it is usually painless. Only a local anesthetic is used, or mild sedation. A small drainage tube can be used to help drain the excess fluids away after surgery. After closing the incision, it is covered with a dressing. The chest might be wrapped to keep the skin firmly in place to promote healing, or a compression garment might be used. The surgery is usually done on an outpatient basis, either in a surgeon's office, outpatient facility, or in some areas, in a hospital.

In severe cases of gynecomastia, sagging excess skin on the breast is removed using an inverted-T or peri-areola breast reduction. In some cases, additional surgery is required to further reduce the size of the areola and nipple or to further lift and reduce the sagging breast skin.

After surgery, expect some pain or discomfort, which is treated with pain medications. Wearing a compression garment can help reduce swelling and should be worn continuously for the first two weeks, and a few weeks longer at night. While the worst swelling disappears after about two weeks, it can take three months or more before the final results of the surgery become apparent.

You can begin walking after a couple of days, and return to work in a week or less. Stitches are removed about two weeks after surgery. You should avoid exercise for three weeks and sex for a week or two. Avoid any activity, like sports, that can cause a blow to the chest for at least four weeks.

As with most plastic surgery, male breast lifts usually are not covered by health insurance plans. However, some plans have reimbursed for the procedure; ask your surgeon's office for help in determining whether you can be reimbursed for your specific surgery. The American Society of Plastic Surgeons has published a white paper defining the recommended criteria for coverage of reconstructive plastic surgery. Your specific case might be covered if your insurance plan honors this documentation.

Neck Lift (Platysmaplasty)

Many obese people carry excess weight in the face and throat area. After massive weight loss, developing a "turkey wattle" (an area of loose, dangling skin, fat and muscle under the chin) is common. Even if other parts of the body become trimmer and tighter, the wattle is a telltale sign that the person was quite heavy at one time.

A neck lift is a procedure that removes excess skin and tightens the underlying muscles if necessary. In many cases, liposuction is also performed. This procedure takes approximately 2-3 hours and is usually done in an outpatient facility using a local anesthetic or mild sedation. If you have other medical issues that put you at higher risk for surgery, it can be performed at a hospital and general anesthesia can be used. It is often done at the same time as a face lift.

Newer procedures have been developed that take only about 1 hour and are much less invasive and less expensive than before, but offer similar results to traditional neck lifts.

Panniculectomy

Excess fat and skin hanging down over the pubic region (a pannicula) is often a feature that most concerns weight-loss patients. Excess skin retains moisture and rashes can result from skin rubbing against itself. To improve contours on the waist back and flanks of weight-loss patients who have lost significant amount of weight, surgeons sometimes perform a belt lipectomy. This incision goes all the way around the patient's midsection at the level just below the waist. These incisions are placed so that the resulting scar is hidden beneath underwear or swimsuits. A panniculectomy removes excess skin and fat but usually does not involve tightening the abdominal muscles, which is done in an abdominoplasty.

Panniculectomies are usually done in hospitals, although some can be done in an outpatient facility. General anesthesia is used and the surgery can require several hours.

Incisions can be horizontal, vertical, or include both. Horizontal incision are usually placed below the underwear line along the pubic bone. Excess skin and fat are removed, and the incisions are closed. Abdominal plastic surgery usually requires drains, which are placed to remove excess fluids from behind the wounds. Dressings are applied and must be kept dry and sterile, and changed as directed.

After surgery, you will be given a list of instructions to follow to avoid complications. Wound care and tending to the drainage tubes is important. Any pain you have can be treated with painkillers. Swelling and bruising are common problems that are manageable. You will not be able to lift more than 5 or 10 pounds for several weeks. You will probably be fitted with a compression garment that must be worn for several weeks after surgery. Many activities are restricted, including sex and exercise, and no pressure can be applied on the abdomen. You will not be able to shower until the incisions have closed and begun to heal, so plan for sponge baths for the first two weeks. Avoid baths, swimming, or soaking in a jacuzzi.

If a panniculectomy is done strictly for cosmetic reasons, it will not be covered by health insurance. However, weight loss patients often have hernias that need repair, which often is covered. Some health insurance plans pay for the whole procedure, while other plans will reimburse for the hernia repair but not the panniculectomy portion of the surgery. If the surgery is done because the excess skin is causing other health problems, such as rashes, soreness or infections, it might be covered. Ask your surgeon's office for help with determining if your health insurance plan will reimburse you for this surgery.

Thigh Lift

There are several types of thigh lifts. An *inner (medial) thigh lift* is performed with an incision in the groin line, lifting the excess skin along the inner part of the thigh and removing the excess skin. The tightening effect extends all the way to the knee. This procedure is less useful if massive weight loss has left significant sagging skin lying on the hipbone area. The incision is considerably smaller than other types of thighplasties, which also limits its usefulness for removing large amounts of skin.

A *vertical thighplasty* involves a vertical incision that extends from the groin line to the inner knee. This procedure reduces the circumference of the leg and is useful for reducing significant excess skin from massive weight loss. The vertical incision can continue further down the leg past the knee to further improve the outcome.

An *outer thigh lift* (*flankoplasty*, *hip lift*) requires an incision that extends from the groin line around the hipbone. It is a modification of an extended abdominoplasty. This procedure is useful because it does not require any scars on the inner thigh and the incision can be placed so that it is covered by clothing. It can be easily combined with an abdominoplasty and done at the same time.

A newer method for an outer thigh lift is called the *spiral thighplasty*, which targets the front, back, inner and outer thigh. The single long incision is made below the fold under the buttocks and continues over the groin crease at the junction of the thigh and pubic area. The buttocks are also lifted. This procedure is effective for people who exhibit a gynoid (pear-shaped) obesity profile.

In many cases, several types of thighplasty are performed at the same time, especially when significant weight that was concentrated in the upper legs is lost.

Either general or twilight anesthesia is used, depending on the extent of the procedure. (With twilight anesthesia, you are sedated but not unconscious.) Liposuction can be used to remove vestiges of fat pockets.

After thigh lift surgery, expect swelling and soreness. Bruising and swelling can be minimized if you take nutritional supplements such as arnica and bromelain before the surgery. There will be some discomfort and tightness for the first two or three days. Painkillers are prescribed for post-surgical pain. The swelling can last up to six weeks. Compression garments are worn to protect the incisions and promote shrinking and tightening of the skin after surgery. Drainage tubes are inserted to reduce swelling and remove excess fluid.

Keep your legs slightly bent at the hips during the first week after surgery to reduce tension on the incision. This produces a thinner, less visible scar. The dressings on your incisions must be kept dry and changed regularly. Do not shower until at least three days after surgery.

Potential Risks and Side Effects

While plastic surgery is often flippantly referred to as a "little nip and tuck," it is in fact a type of surgery that has significant impact.

A significant commitment is required to have bariatric surgery and then lose the required weight over an 18 month period, which is then followed by the body contouring surgeries and recovery. This process can take three years from beginning to end.

Plastic surgery has many of the same risks as bariatric surgery. For more information, see "Potential Problems or Complications After Weight Loss Surgery" on page 119.

Risks associated with plastic surgery also include:

✓ infection

✓ scarring

✓ bleeding

✓ reaction to medications

✓ reactions to or complications of anesthesia

✓ pain

✓ nausea

✓ swelling and bruising

✓ sutures that poke through the skin, becoming visible or causing irritation that requires removal

✓ fat necrosis

✓ allergic reactions to dressings, sutures, glue, blood products, or injections

✓ deep vein thrombosis, cardiac and pulmonary complications

The process for body contouring (specifically a full body lift) can require seven to ten hours under general anesthesia, blood transfusions, and often requires a team of surgeons to complete a single operation. For example, a panniculectomy is often done by two surgeons, one working on each side of the body.

Because blood transfusions are often used for this type of extensive surgery, many patients use *autologous* (self-donated) blood. For several weeks before surgery, pints of your blood are withdrawn, frozen and stored for surgery. If blood products are needed during the surgery, your own blood can be used, avoiding the risk of blood-transmitted diseases.

Most cosmetic surgeons discourage weight loss surgery patients who have not yet lost 50% of their excess weight from having body contouring surgery. These surgeries are not a type of obesity operation.

Additionally, many weight loss patients have had co-morbid conditions over a long period of time that can contribute to outcomes that are less than successful. These include heart disease or bleeding disorders. If you smoke, your surgical risk is considerably higher. Scars already on the body can cause problems for cosmetic surgeons.

You can develop *seroma*, a pocket of clear or pink serous fluid that develops after surgery. It consists of blood plasma leaking from small blood vessels that were cut or ruptured. Inflammation caused by dying injured cells often contributes to the serous fluid, along with liquefied fats from dead fat cells. The excess fluid that causes swelling of the tissues is also part of the seroma. Seromas are different from *hematomas*, which contain red blood cells, and *abscesses*, which contain pus generated by an infection. Seroma is common after cosmetic or abdominal surgery.

Some people can also have *dehiscence* (wound separation) or *deep vein thrombosis* (blood clots that form in the legs). Wound separations are usually small and minor, but if it occurs, consult your plastic surgeon to see if further treatment is needed.

Changes in skin sensation that causes numbness after surgery are common. Some sensation usually returns over the three to eight months after surgery, but the area might not return to the same level of sensitivity as before the surgery and can become hypersensitive in some people. The area can become itchy or tender, or become very sensitive to temperature changes. These effects are usually short lived and can be managed with moisturizers, medication and massage.

Your navel, which is repositioned during abdominal plastic surgery, might be slightly asymmetrical or off-center.

Asymmetry after any plastic surgery is always a possibility. Most people have asymmetric bodies before surgery; while a plastic surgeon takes great care to ensure symmetry, your left and right sides might not be an exact mirror image after surgery. It is possible that this will be permanent, due to skeletal bone prominence, fatty deposits, muscle development or skin tone that cannot be corrected with plastic surgery.

After abdominoplasty, body lifts and thigh lifts, the pubic area can appear distorted, since the skin in this area is lifted and flattened during these procedures. It can range from minor distortion that improves naturally over time to a problem that cannot be corrected. It does not occur generally.

Our two perpetual enemies – age and gravity – will cause additional lack of firmness and mild sagging in the future. However, the results you see one to two years after your plastic surgery should be permanent, as long as you do not gain a significant amount of weight. You should also plan on maintaining an exercise and diet plan for the rest of your life to maintain your new body.

What About Scars and Pain?

Scars from plastic surgery appear to look worse over the first weeks or months after surgery. It can take up to 18 months before they flatten and lighten in color. While the scars never disappear, they can usually be hidden by clothing.

You can reduce scars by applying a topical steroid skin cream for 4 to 6 weeks following surgery. The scars fade faster and become much less noticeable. These skin creams can be found in any drugstore.

Some patients become nauseous after anesthesia. Nausea is often caused by pain. To reduce this effect, you might be prescribed Decadron (a steroid used to reduce nausea), Zofran (an anti-nausea medication often prescribed for cancer patients) and Pepcid AC (an over-the-counter medication which inhibits nausea). You might also be prescribed additional pain medications whose side effects include the tendency to reduce nausea and vomiting.

11

Potential Problems or Complications After Weight Loss Surgery

A number of potential problems can occur after weight loss surgery. Some problems are related to the surgery itself and are usually seen immediately during the first one or two weeks after the surgery is performed. Others are long-term issues that can continue to develop for several years after surgery.

Statistically, 10 to 20% of all bariatric patients develop a complication that requires additional surgery to correct, with hernias the most common problem, followed by gallstones.

It is important to remember that after bariatric surgery, **any** abdominal pain must not be ignored. If you suspect a problem, contact your bariatric surgeon immediately.

Complications Related To Co-morbid Conditions

Bariatric surgery has been shown to help resolve or cure many obesity health-related conditions. However, just having some of the co-morbid conditions that are often improved after surgery can increase your risk for developing complications.

✓ Patients with higher body mass index (BMI) have an increased risk of complications. To reduce this risk, your bariatric surgeon probably required you to begin losing weight before surgery. Pre-surgical weight loss also has the benefit of reducing internal fat stored inside the abdominal cavity. Excess internal abdominal fat makes the surgical procedure more difficult to perform, because it limits accessibility to the internal organs.

✓ High blood pressure before surgery can increase problems with blood clotting after surgery.

✓ If you had previous problems with deep vein thrombosis in the arms or legs, pulmonary embolism, or other blood clotting problems in the past, your risk for experiencing them after bariatric surgery is increased.

✓ Sleep apnea, diabetes and arthritis increase your chances for developing *sepsis* (the presence of pus-forming bacteria or their toxins in the blood).

✓ Sleep apnea and gastroesophageal reflux disease (GERD) result in the highest risk for bariatric surgery complications.

✓ Any obesity-related health problem before surgery increases your risk of complications. You have a 27.5% higher risk of developing dumping syndrome, a 24.5% increased chance of developing complications related to the anastomosis, and a 23.5% higher chance of developing sepsis.[1]

Restrictive procedures, like gastric band surgery or vertical banded gastroplasty, have surgical complications that are similar to malabsorptive procedures.

Weight Loss Surgery and Food Addictions

A study that was aired on the Oprah Winfrey show October 24, 2006 claimed that 30% of people who undergo weight loss surgery suffer from an addiction transference, which is transferring the previous addiction to food into an addiction to alcohol.

There have been no scientific studies that prove this theory, and its basis is doubted by many people in the medical profession. There is also an absence of any anecdotal evidence needed to support it.

---

1   J Cawley, et al. Predicting Complications after Bariatric Surgery using Obesity-Related Co-morbidities. Obesity Surgery." November 2007. Vol 17, Num 11. Pgs 1451-1456.

Bariatric surgery does not cure food addiction. Fortunately, many of the foods that are so enticing before surgery — foods containing fats, sugars or carbohydrates — become less enticing after surgery, particularly if you have one of the malabsorptive procedures. People who are addicted to sweets, for example, who have Roux-en-Y surgery often develop dumping syndrome, a condition that results in moderate or severe discomfort, if they ingest these types of foods. People who are addicted to fatty foods who have biliopancreatic diversion with duodenal switch surgery often find their tolerance level to fats is greatly reduced after surgery. Complications like diarrhea or a number of loose stools each day tend to discourage the consumption of more fats.

Restrictive procedures, on the other hand, can only limit the amount of food consumed at one time. Those who routinely do not stop eating after having normal portions can benefit from restrictive surgery. The food addiction is not cured, but it becomes significantly more difficult to accommodate.

Short Term Problems Following Surgery

Problems such as bleeding and infection are seen after many types of surgeries, not just weight loss surgeries.

Bleeding

In bariatric surgery (other than gastric banding), many blood vessels are cut when the stomach is divided and the small intestine is moved. Any of these can begin to bleed into the abdominal cavity (*intra-abdominal hemorrhage*) or into the intestinal tract (*gastrointestinal hemorrhage*).

If bleeding is severe, blood transfusions might be required, along with additional surgery to repair the damaged blood vessel.

Patients who are on blood thinner therapy have an increased risk of bleeding. The blood thinners are discontinued before surgery and not restarted for several days or weeks until the danger of spontaneous bleeding is reduced. In some cases, weight loss patients are medicated with blood thinners to prevent pulmonary embolism, which slightly increases the risk of bleeding. If you take blood thinners, dosage and blood levels must be carefully and frequently monitored to avoid problems. Because bleeding problems can develop at any time, this visual inspection should continue for the rest of your life.

Blackened stools can indicate a bleeding problem. While some people are squeamish about it, you should visually inspect your stools before flushing to catch any bleeding problems early.

Wound Infections

Infections of the incisions or of the internal abdominal wall can cause peritonitis or abscess, which are caused by bacteria that are released from the intestinal tract during the surgery.

Nosocomial infections, which include pneumonia, bladder or kidney infections, occur infrequently as the result of treatment in a hospital or health care facility. Septic (blood borne) infections can also occur.

The risk of infection can be reduced after surgery by following antiseptic techniques, increased physical activity, diligent pulmonary therapy (deep breathing) done every hour, and the use of antibiotics.

Blood Clots (Pulmonary Embolism)

A pulmonary embolism is a blood clot that forms elsewhere in the body and moves into the lungs, affecting less than 1% of all bariatric surgery patients. However, developing pulmonary embolisms is a serious issue – they are the major cause of death after weight loss surgery.

Blood clots can be prevented by using blood thinning prescription medications like Warfarin, or by ensuring you get enough exercise after surgery. Patients are routinely told to begin walking within a few hours after surgery (as long as they can stand without falling). Some surgeons start their patients on prophylactic doses of 81mg enteric aspirin as a preventive measure. Your surgeon might also require you to wear elastic compression stockings while lying in bed, or prescribe the use of inflatable stockings which rhythmically compress in a way that moves blood out of the legs and back towards the heart.

It is essential to continue moving as much as possible after you are released from the hospital to avoid pulmonary embolism.

Symptoms include shortness of breath, chest pain and coughing. Other symptoms include wheezing, swelling in the legs, clammy or bluish-colored skin, excessive sweating, rapid or irregular heartbeat, weak pulse and feeling light-headed or fainting. If you develop any of these symptoms, consult your surgeon immediately. A pulmonary embolism can be life-threatening if immediate action is not taken.

Dysphagia (Difficulty in Swallowing)

Dysphagia is a medical term for difficulty in swallowing. Dysphagia is a side effect of any bariatric surgery that involves restriction (including Roux-en-Y, biliopancreatic diversion with duodenal switch, and gastric band). It is caused by eating too quickly, eating too much, or not chewing enough before swallowing after the stomach has been made smaller.

After gastric band surgery, the extra food cannot pass the band stricture quickly enough, so it stays in the lower esophagus and eventually causes the esophagus to stretch and expand, acting like an additional stomach that enables more food to be ingested.

Symptoms of dysphagia include pressure in the chest or tightness in the throat.

Dysphagia can be reduced or eliminated by chewing food 15 or more times before swallowing, by slowing ingestion (by putting your fork down for one minute between bites), and avoiding tough foods like overcooked steaks or doughy breads. Remember to consult with your bariatric surgeon before you make changes in your diet.

If you had gastric band surgery and had the band tightened, you might notice symptoms of dysphagia. To avoid this, follow a liquid diet for two days after band tightening, followed by two days of soft foods and progression to solid foods on the fifth day after the tightening. If you cannot get used to the new level of tightness after a week, the band can be loosened again.

Esophageal dilation can also indicate that the band was improperly placed, which would require revisional surgery to place the band in the correct location.

Treatment usually involves loosening the gastric band slightly, along with reducing the quantity of food ingested. Eating softer foods is often helpful, as is slowing down when you eat. More severe cases can require removal of the band.

Dysphagia can be commonly seen for about six months after bariatric surgery, improving slowly as the anastomosis stretches. Suffering from extreme dysphagia four to six weeks after surgery or difficulty in drinking fluids can indicate an anastomotic stricture, which can be treated endoscopically. For more information, see "Anastomotic Stricture" on page 145.

Anastomotic Leaks

Anastomotic leaks can occur in Roux-en-Y and biliopancreatic diversion with duodenal switch surgeries. An *anastomosis* is the surgical connection between the stomach and bowel or between two parts of the bowel. The connection is made using staples or sutures, both of which make holes in the wall of the bowel. As the body heals, scar tissue is formed that seals the connection and makes it watertight, in much the same way as a self-sealing tire works.

If the seal is not watertight, fluids from the intestinal tract can leak into the normally sterile abdominal cavity, causing infections or abscesses which can lead to peritonitis or death.

Anastomotic leakage, usually at the stomach to bowel connection, occurs in about 2% of Roux-en-Y and biliopancreatic diversion with duodenal switch surgeries.

Anastomotic leakage is usually discovered after an infection or abscess has developed and begins to cause pain. It should be treated immediately; it can be life-threatening.

Minor leakage can be treated with antibiotics. If it cannot be controlled quickly, corrective surgery is performed to reconnect the stomach and bowel.

Staple Failure

The staples that are routinely used in bariatric surgery to reduce the size of the stomach can pull loose. This is almost always avoidable and is related to eating too much food after surgery. People who constantly feel very full after eating or who have stomach discomfort related to food intake should be especially careful.

Staple failure can lead to the acidic contents of the stomach leaking into the abdominal cavity, which affects nearby organs and can cause infection or death.

You should never eat so much food that you feel too full or significantly uncomfortable after eating. Post-surgical bariatric patients must master portion size control.

Temporary Hair Loss

Patients who have had malabsorptive surgical procedures can suffer temporary hair loss. It is a result of inadequate protein intake and can be complicated by vitamin deficiencies. All bariatric patients should expect to lose some hair, but you will not go bald. Hair loss is related primarily to unmet nutritional needs and is known as *telogen effluvium*. The condition often resolves as time passes and if nutritional needs are met.

Fear of hair loss is the reason why the majority of female patients delay having their bariatric surgery. Ironically, in surveys done before surgery, many obese people point to their hair as their best feature.

Hair loss often begins to become noticeable four or five months after surgery. This is the period when caloric input is at its lowest. Your pre-surgical diet was probably 3,000 calories a day or more; after surgery, it can be as little as 500 or 600 calories a day. While a normal body sheds about 10% of its hair at any time, a body that thinks it is facing starvation will drop thirty or forty percent of its hair as the body channels what little nutrients it is receiving to more vital areas, like the internal organs and muscles. In addition to hair that is shed, the remaining hair becomes dull and lifeless.

Hair follicles have two states: *anagen* and *telogen*. During the anagen stage, hair is living and growing. In the telogen stage, the hair follicle dies and falls out. At any point in time, 90% of your hair is anagen and 10% is telogen, which means that we constantly add more hair than we lose. After a hair follicle enters the telogen phase, it is dead and will not go back to an anagen state. So, no matter what miracle hair cure you use, nothing can revive a dead telogen follicle and make it continue to grow and thrive.

In addition to nutritional deficiencies, hair loss is caused by a number of other reasons, including major surgery, high fever, severe infection, and so forth. Bariatric patients have both major surgery and nutritional causes, along with other causes that vary by individual.

Hair loss is resolved when your weight stabilizes and your nutritional needs are met through diet and supplementation. Several vitamins can help with healthy hair growth.

In the meantime, avoid well-intended "remedies" that can actually cause the problem to worsen:

✓ avoid hair bands, barrettes, scarves, and hats — anything that pulls on the hair follicles in the scalp

✓ avoid hairstyles that involve teasing or elaborate combing

✓ avoid hot rollers, hair dryers or hot curlers

✓ if you color your hair, do it less frequently, if at all, during this period

✓ permanents can make hair brittle and are best avoided

✓ use this opportunity to try new hair styles that are shorter, uncurled, and uncolored

✓ short hair falls out less than very long hair

✓ switch to a shampoo that is very mild, like baby shampoo, or one that contains nioxin

Scalp massage, which promotes blood flow to the scalp, can be helpful. Brushing your hair does the same thing, but it also stresses the hair by pulling on it. Scalp massage, if done correctly, does not involve pulling on the hair.

Be sure to include iron supplements if you are losing hair. While iron deficiency often results in anemia, you can still develop a non-anemic iron deficiency. Blood tests performed by your bariatric surgeon or primary care physician can determine if you need more iron supplementation.

Hair loss can also indicate a zinc deficiency. A topical preparation of zinc sulfate has been used in clinical research studies, with decent results.[2]

---

2   H Neve, W Bhatti, C Soulsby, et al. "Reversal of hair loss following vertical gastroplasty when treated with zinc sulphate." Obesity Surgery. Vol 199:6(1). Pgs 63–65.

Protein deficiency can contribute to hair loss.[3] Hair is made of protein and is susceptible to nutritional protein deficiency. Research has indicated a link between an amino acid called l-lysine; supplementing with lysine has been related to regrowth of healthy hair follicles in study participants.[4, 5]

Many people use biotin supplements (Vitamin B7, also known as Vitamin H) to combat hair loss. It can be consumed in tablet form, or applied topically as a powder on the scalp. To date, there are no conclusive studies that show the effectiveness of biotin, but several bariatric patients I know insist it has helped with their hair loss issues in the absence of any other remedies.

You can also try applying special shampoos and oils, such as shampoo with nioxin and flax seed oil.

Some bariatric patients also use Silica, a supplement that helps hair and nail growth. There are no conclusive studies that verify this, but it is generally used as a supplement with good results.

Thrush (Yeast Infection)

If you take antibiotics after surgery to prevent infection, you can develop a yeast infection of the mouth called *thrush*. Symptoms include changes of the tongue, such as a white coating, redness or inflammation.

Thrush is easily treated with medication. If you develop these symptoms, consult your physician.

Problems That Develop Over Time

As time passes after bariatric surgery, additional issues arise that can require treatment. Some begin early on, while others do not develop until some time passes after surgery.

---

3   V Moize, A Geliebter, ME Gluck, et al. "Obese patients have inadequate protein intake related to protein intolerance up to 1 year following Roux-en-Y gastric bypass." Obesity Surgery. 2003; Vol 13:1. Pgs 23–28.

4   Ibid.

5   TA Updegraff, NJ Neufeld. "Protein, iron, and folate status of patients prior to and following surgery for morbid obesity." Journal of the American Dietary Association. 1981. Volume 78 Issue 2. Pages 135–140.

Dyspepsia (Indigestion)

Indigestion is a fact of life after all forms of bariatric surgery. After altering the digestive tract, the body has to learn how to handle food digestion tasks that no longer fit the norm. Some period of compensation in the form of indigestive upset is seen after all types of bariatric surgery. As time passes, the body becomes acclimated to the anatomical changes and symptoms of indigestion are reduced.

Symptoms include an uncomfortable sensation in the abdomen after eating, nausea, or vomiting.

This period of indigestion has a beneficial aspect. If certain foods make you feel ill, you won't want to continue eating them. The good news is that the foods which cause the most digestive upset are the same foods (sugars, carbohydrates and fatty foods) that should be avoided for optimal weight loss after surgery.

Ulcers

Stomal ulcers are acid-peptic ulcers that develop at or near the anastomosis (the surgically-created connection between stomach pouch and intestine). An ulcer can also develop in the intestinal tract itself.

The risk for developing ulcers increases after bariatric surgery. Between 5 and 15% of bariatric patients report symptoms of ulcers. Patients who use non-steroid anti-inflammatory drugs (NSAIDs) and smokers have an even higher risk. For this reason, all post-bariatric patients are advised to avoid NSAIDs, such as Advil, Aleve, Haltran, Midol, Motrin and Nuprin, after surgery and for the rest of their lives, and to abstain from smoking.

Ulcers can lead to erosion of gastric bands into the stomach wall, so gastric band patients should also avoid NSAIDs.

Constipation

You can develop constipation after bariatric surgery. It is often seen in gastric band surgeries, and less frequently after Roux-en-Y and biliopancreatic diversion with duodenal switch surgeries. Constipation results from an inadequate intake of fluids, especially water. Increasing water consumption can help in treatment, along with adding fiber products (like Metamucil or Fibercon) or high-fiber foods.

It is helpful to avoid diuretics and caffeine. Some pain medications can also interfere with bowel function, resulting in constipation.

In many cases, nutritional supplements like iron and calcium can contribute to problems with constipation. If you become constipated while taking nutritional supplements, adding a stool softener can help. Avoid stool softener products that also contain laxatives to avoid becoming laxative-dependent.

Hernia

A hernia is an abnormal opening within the abdomen or in the abdominal wall.

Internal hernias occur after surgery and rearrangement of the bowel. This form of hernia can easily become obstructed.

Incisional hernias occur when the abdominal wall muscles do not heal well, allowing the muscle fibers to separate and a sac-like membrane to protrude through the opening. This sac can contain portions of bowel or other abdominal components and is often unsightly as well as being painful. Newer types of weight loss surgery that use laparoscopic methods result in fewer hernias, because the organs inside the abdominal cavity are too large to pass through such small incisions.

Some hernias do not need further treatment, while larger hernias or those involving abdominal organs are often corrected surgically. This becomes essential if the hernia becomes twisted or strangulated and restricts the contents of the bowel from passing through it. Severe and sudden pain in the abdomen can indicate a hernia. If this occurs, consult your bariatric surgeon immediately.

Gallstones

Rapid weight loss can cause the formation of cholesterol gallstones. This condition is so widespread among bariatric post-surgical patients that many bariatric surgeons routinely remove the gall bladder during the bariatric surgery.

Developing gallstones is more likely in the six month period following the bariatric surgery. This is the time when the most weight is quickly lost. As time progresses, weight loss continues, but at a slower rate. More than 33% of all bariatric patients, regardless of whether their surgery was restrictive, malabsorptive or a combination, develop gallstones.

It is not helpful that obese people have a much higher rate of gallstone formation than the normal population. By age 50, about 50% of morbidly obese women have developed gallstones.

Many surgeons prescribe bile salts, a medication that helps prevent the formation of gallstones, to be taken as a preventive measure after surgery.

If your gall bladder must be removed surgically, it is often done laparoscopically.

Excess Skin

After bariatric surgery, fat cells can be shed so rapidly that the stretched skin cannot contract quickly enough.

Because weight loss after gastric band surgery occurs at a slower rate than other bariatric surgeries, this problem is often less severe after gastric band.

There are several ways to reduce excess loose skin, or plastic surgery can be used to eliminate it. These options are discussed in "Plastic Surgery" on page 89.

Skin Problems

Dermatological problems, such as acne or dry skin, occur with some bariatric patients. They are often a result of a nutritional deficiency. Following a bariatric diet and taking nutritional supplements can be helpful. Ointments, lotions and medications that are available over the counter can be used as necessary. For severe conditions, or dermatological conditions that do not resolve within a few days, consult a dermatologist.

Calmoseptine® is a moisture barrier ointment that is available over-the-counter to alleviate skin discomfort and itching. Originally used as a diaper ointment, it is effective for relieving the discomfort from moist, irritated skin. Ointments containing titanium dioxide are useful, as are those traditionally used for diaper rash.

Avoid tight-fitting clothing that can chafe the skin. Elastic bands can contribute to skin irritation.

Feeling Cold

After surgery, and as you lose more weight, you might notice that you feel cold. This occurs for two reasons: your metabolism changes after surgery as your weight drops, and there is less body fat to insulate you from outside temperatures.

For many of those who have been significantly overweight for much of their lives, the sensation of feeling cold is both strange and welcome.

Gurgling Noises in the Abdomen

Many bariatric patients report an increase in loud gurgling noises in the abdomen. This is caused by the way your new digestive system pushes air through the intestinal tract.

Other than noises, which can be relatively loud and somewhat embarrassing, there is usually no discomfort or other symptoms.

To reduce abdominal gurgling, do not:

✓ consume fizzy drinks (carbonated beverages)

✓ drink through a straw

✓ chew gum

✓ suck on hard candy

✓ eat or drink too quickly

Many people develop a habit of eating too quickly and swallowing air rapidly in order to produce a belch to relieve the discomfort caused by eating too fast. This can become an unconscious habit. After surgery, even small amounts of excess air can cause abdominal gurgling.

Dumping Syndrome

The function of the pyloric valve at the base of the human stomach is to open and close to deliver amounts of food gradually into the duodenum. The stomach, liver and pancreas work together to prepare nutrients (primarily sugars) before they reach the small intestine for absorption. The stomach is a type of reservoir, releasing food downstream at a controlled rate to avoid large discharges of sugar into the intestinal tract. The food that is released is mixed with acids from the stomach, bile from the liver, and pancreatic juice to control the chemical balance and composition of the food being moved downstream.

Dumping Syndrome occurs only with Roux-en-Y patients because that surgery involves bypassing the pyloric valve. About 85% of Roux-en-Y patients experience dumping syndrome. Symptoms can range from mild to severe.

There are two forms of dumping: early dumping and late dumping.

Early dumping syndrome happens when the lower end of the intestine (the jejunum) fills too quickly with undigested food from the stomach. The duodenum expands too quickly as the undigested food is pushed through it. The body floods the bowel with extra fluids in an attempt to dilute the partly–digested sugars, which irritate the jejunum.

Symptoms of early dumping syndrome include abdominal pain or cramping, bloating, vomiting, sweating, flushing, rapid heart rate or palpitations, feeling light-headed, upper abdominal fullness, nausea and audible bowel sounds. Many patients have diarrhea. Symptoms are noted 30 to 60 minutes after eating.

Late dumping syndrome is related to blood sugar levels. The small intestine is very efficient in absorbing sugars, so the rapid absorption of even small amounts of sugar can cause the glucose level in the blood to rise rapidly. The pancreas responds to the excess glucose by increasing insulin output. The amount of sugar that started the process was so relatively small that it does not maintain the higher glucose levels, which begin to fall at about the same time as the increased insulin is released. This produces hypoglycemia (low blood sugar). This type of hypoglycemia is called *alimentary hypoglycemia*.

The symptoms of late dumping syndrome include feeling weak, sleepy or fatigued, sweating, shakiness, loss of concentration, hunger or passing out.

One problem associated with late dumping syndrome is that the patient often feels hungry again shortly after experiencing the dumping. This is due to the excess insulin in the bloodstream, which triggers feelings of hunger. It becomes easy to fall into a cycle of eating more food simply because you feel hungry again.

The best treatment for early dumping syndrome is to avoid the foods that cause it. Avoid simple sugars. Restricting high glycemic carbohydrates, such as potatoes, pasta, or other sweet-tasting foods) is often helpful, as is eating more protein and fiber, which move more slowly from the stomach pouch.

If treating the early dumping syndrome does not work, late dumping syndrome can be treated by taking a small amount of sugar, such as a few ounces of orange juice, about an hour after eating. Medications are also available to treat late dumping syndrome if dietary changes are ineffective.

Drink liquids between meals, not with them, to slow the progression of food out of the stomach. Food that is very hot or very cold can also trigger symptoms of dumping syndrome.

Following a balanced diet is important. People with dumping syndrome need to eat several smaller meals a day to maintain their blood sugar levels. You should avoid simple sugars. Medications can be used to slow the digestive process. Revisional surgery can sometimes be performed to change the routing of the intestinal tract to lessen the symptoms, although this is not frequently done.

Dumping syndrome has both positive and negative aspects. Most bariatric surgeons consider dumping syndrome to be a benefit of bariatric surgery. It provides a quick and reliable negative reinforcement mechanism when food choices are poor. When you eat the wrong types of foods and develop dumping syndrome, you are less likely to eat that food again. You quickly learn which foods can be tolerated and to avoid the ones that cause discomfort. The foods that cause dumping are the same ones that interfere with long–term weight loss success. Many post-surgery patients report that after suffering even a few bouts of dumping syndrome, they find that they have lost their craving for sweets.

Bowel Obstruction

The process of cutting into the intestines and subsequent scarring can cause bowel obstructions called *adhesions*. A hernia, either internal or through the abdominal wall, can also occur.

When a section of the intestine becomes entrapped by adhesions or hernia, it can kink and become obstructed. This can occur many years after the surgery. The loss of internal abdominal fat, which can serve to keep the internal organs in place, can also contribute to hernia by allowing the intestines to move slightly. This is more likely after abdominal surgery where the intestines have been handled or cut.

Surgery is usually required to correct a bowel obstruction. Because an obstructed bowel can be very painful, it is usually quickly diagnosed and resolved.

Diarrhea and Loose Stools (Steatorrhea)

Bariatric surgeries make permanent changes to the gastrointestinal tract. Bowel function is often altered. The issues that result can be short-term or long-term, and range from mild to severe. Changes that are short-term are relatively easy to manage. Chronic issues can need management over a long period of time or for the rest of the patient's life.

Diarrhea is a potential side effect in both Roux-en-Y and biliopancreatic diversion with duodenal switch surgeries. It is not noted in people who had gastric band surgeries.

Diarrhea and loose stools are often related to the diet. Avoiding foods that trigger the condition is the best defense.

Roux-en-Y and biliopancreatic diversion with duodenal switch patients have had forms of duodenal switch. Diarrhea is caused by the release of fatty acids directly into the colon that normally would have been absorbed in the small intestine. With a significant length of the small intestine bypassed, the fatty acids do not have the opportunity to become absorbed. Diarrhea is also produced when partly digested food is passed into the gastrointestinal tract. It also is a side effect of sorbitol, an artificial sweetener that is also found naturally in fruits and berries and in many sugar-free foods. Sorbitol is not well absorbed in the gastrointestinal tract, and when it reaches the colon, it ferments. This fermentation process produces excess foul-smelling gas and diarrhea.

Some people who had surgeries that included a duodenal switch have two or three bowel movements a day, although a small percentage report a much higher number (between 10 and 20 per day). Most patients return to a single bowel movement a day.

Diarrhea can usually be controlled by altering the diet. Reducing the amount of fats is helpful. Diarrhea can also indicate that the entire diet needs to be monitored and adjusted. Certain foods trigger diarrhea in specific individuals; those foods should be avoided or minimized.

Many bariatric patients are prescribed *probiotics*, a form of colonic bacteria that exist normally in humans. Additional probiotics are ingested to increase the amount of these bacteria to help with the digestive process. You can also buy foods, such as yogurts, that have probiotic cultures already added.

If diarrhea continues for more than a year after surgery, revisional surgery can be performed to lengthen the common channel of the bowel. This surgery is usually relatively uncomplicated and can be done laparoscopically, requiring only an overnight stay in the hospital. The diarrhea should resolve after surgery, with no subsequent weight gain.

Gas and Bloating

In the unaltered anatomy, the stomach begins the digestive process and then moves the contents into the duodenum, where it is broken down with enzymes and more completely digested.

In the altered anatomy after bariatric surgery (other than gastric band surgery), the stomach does not act on its contents as it did in the past. Partly digested food is released into the gastrointestinal tract at a point that in unaltered anatomy is much further along the tract. The gastric juices and the enzymes produced and acted upon in the duodenum do not have the time to digest the food properly, resulting in food moving through the gastrointestinal tract that is only partly digested. When acted upon by bacteria in the colon, it ferments and creates gas.

Excess gas is caused by the types of food you consume.

Sugars are often to blame. Consuming too much lactose can cause problems, as can fructose and sorbitol. *Lactose* is found in milk and milk products, and in bread, cereal and salad dressings. *Fructose* is found in pears, onions and wheat, among others, and is used as a sweetener in soft drinks and fruit drinks. *Raffinose*, which is contained in beans, cabbage, brussels sprouts, broccoli, asparagus and other vegetables, also causes gas and bloating. *Sorbitol* is found in fruits like pears, apples, peaches and prunes, and is used as an artificial sweetener in dietetic foods and sugar-free candies and chewing gums. Sorbitol is a major ingredient in baby laxatives.

Carbohydrates (starches) also can cause gas and bloating. Potatoes, corn, pasta and wheat all cause gas as they are broken down in the digestive tract. Rice, however, does not create excess gas or bloating.

There are two forms of fiber. *Soluble fiber* dissolves easily in water and takes on a gelatinous texture in the gastrointestinal tract. Soluble fiber is found in oat bran, beans, peas and most fruits, and it does not break down until it reaches the large intestine, where digestion causes gas and bloating.

Insoluble fiber, found in wheat bran and some vegetables, does not break down at all and does not cause gas. You can adjust your diet to eliminate much of the soluble fiber and increase the amount of insoluble fiber.

Many people swallow excess air when they eat. Normally, the result is an occasional belch, or the air becomes incorporated in the swallowed food and moves along the gastrointestinal tract. You can also swallow excess air if you drink through a straw, suck on hard candy or chew gum. You can reduce or eliminate these habits if gas becomes problematic.

For most people, eating fewer foods that cause gas and bloating relieves the condition. However, for bariatric patients, this can mean eliminating foods that are otherwise healthy from your diet.

Fats and proteins cause very little gas, so they are usually not a problem in the post-surgical diet.

Each person's diet is different, and each body processes food differently. Finding the correct balance as you make changes in your diet is done through trial and error.

Digestive enzymes, available over the counter in drugstores, can be used to help digest carbohydrates. Lactase tablets are available to help with lactose digestion. Milk products are available with the digestive enzyme already added (Lactaid) at grocery stores. Beano tablets can help with digestion of sugars found in beans and other vegetables. Products like Gas-X can also be used to reduce excess gas. If your tendency towards gas and bloating is diagnosed to be caused by *Irritable Bowel Syndrome* (IBS), your physician can prescribe medication that can help. These medications are helpful if the gas is produced by specific conditions in the body, but are not usually used if excess gas is caused only by diet.

Flatulence

Excessive flatulence is one relatively unpublicized side effect after malabsorptive bariatric surgeries. Not only is excess gas produced — sometimes a lot of excess gas — but it is also highly malodorous. It is generally not as great a problem in procedures that are only restrictive, like gastric band.

The malabsorptive quality of Roux-en-Y and biliopancreatic diversion with duodenal switch surgeries prevents the digestive system from absorbing the food and nutrients as well as it did before. When the undigested food is pushed into the colon, enzymes and bacteria are produced to digest the food. One of their by-products is excess gas.

Many post-surgical bariatric patients are embarrassed by their flatulence; many of them have been dealing with embarrassment throughout much of their lives. Most of them try various over the counter medications, many of which are ineffective.

Certain foods, such as carbohydrates, are acknowledged to cause flatulence. Reducing the intake of these foods can help alleviate the problem, but it is rarely completely resolved. Each patient has different needs, so you might have to experiment with your own diet to find out which foods seem to trigger flatulence. Often certain types of foods, like cruciform vegetables (for example, cauliflower, broccoli and cabbage) create more hydrogen sulfide during the digestive process than other foods. Hydrogen sulfide is the primary chemical that causes malodorous flatulence.

Devrom is an over-the-counter oral medication that is often prescribed to reduce the odors associated with flatulence. Weight loss surgery patients have reported varying levels of effectiveness: the medication works well for some people and not at all for others. Since it is easily available without a prescription, it is worth trying to see if it will work for you.

Taking activated charcoal tablets has been helpful in many cases. The charcoal is an inert substance that absorbs odors and passes easily through the system.

As the number of post-surgical bariatric patients increases, solutions are being marketed to help with the problem. Several companies offer activated charcoal products to help absorb odors, including Flat-D and

GasBGon. They are available as pads (resembling sanitary napkins but much less bulky) that are inserted in the underwear. One type is worn for a day and then discarded; another type is reusable. They are available in various thicknesses to accommodate different needs. The company also makes activated charcoal seat pads for chairs (including office chairs). The pads have been used over a number of years by ostomy patients, who have the same issues of malodorous gas and flatulence.

Lactose Intolerance

Lactose is a sugar that occurs naturally in cow milk products. It is digested in the stomach by the enzyme lactase. About 10% of Americans are lactose intolerant, and about 50% of the world's population suffers from it. After bariatric surgery, the smaller stomach pouch cannot produce as much lactase as an intact stomach, and bariatric patients frequently discover that they have become lactose intolerant. In the smaller stomachs of bariatric patients, milk products also move quickly into the intestinal tract while the lactose in the milk is still undigested.

Many bariatric surgeons believe that gastric bypass surgeries can reveal pre-existing lactose intolerance, but not cause it directly. Others attribute it directly to the surgical changes made to the stomach, specifically the reduction of availability of mucosal tissue that manufacturers lactase in the section of the stomach that was bypassed.

Symptoms include cramps or abdominal pain, bloating, gas, nausea and diarrhea. The symptoms can be variable; it is not unusual to be more or less lactose intolerant on different days, at different times of the day and as the diet varies.

The problem with any disorder that causes diarrhea is that the condition reduces the amount of nutrition your body can extract from the foods you eat. After bariatric surgery, any food that you eat should be contributing towards your good health and maintaining vigor.

Bariatric patients can reduce their intake of milk and milk products, ingest them more slowly or eat thicker or processed milk products like cheeses and yogurts instead of liquid milk. You might have to avoid milk products completely to eliminate the symptoms if you are significantly lactose intolerant.

Many products on the grocery shelves contain milk products, including hot dogs, cold cuts, candy, cookies, bread, commercial sauces and gravies, dessert mixes, cereals, frosting, salad dressings, cream soups and even medications. Post-bariatric patients quickly learn to read package labels to see both ingredient lists and nutritional data.

You can also take an enzyme substitute (Lactaid) with milk products. The enzyme is available in tablet and liquid forms. Milk products with the enzyme already added are available at the grocery store.

Stomal Stenosis

Stomal stenosis is the narrowing of the outlet between the stomach pouch and the small intestine. It occurs because the scar tissue that forms at the surgical site tightens and shrinks over time. It can shrink to the point where it begins to prevent the passage of food from the stomach. It occurs in 5 to 15% of bariatric surgeries in which the duodenum is separated and reattached. If this happens, a corrective surgery can be performed to enlarge the anastomosis.

Symptoms include vomiting and nausea after eating.

Most patients eat enough bulky food so that the process of stretching the scar tissue happens at a rate equal to the shrinkage rate, and the anastomosis remains at an adequate size.

Food Blockage

The smaller passageway between stomach and gastrointestinal tract after a restrictive weight loss surgery can cause occasional food blockage. This is often caused by eating food too fast or by not chewing food enough.

The symptoms of food blockage are an uncomfortable feeling in the pit of the stomach, vomiting or retching.

The food usually dissolves by itself, or the weight of incoming food pushes it through the opening and out of the stomach. Vomiting can often dislodge the food from the anastomosis. In severe cases, an endoscopic procedure can be used to clear the food blockage.

Hyperparathyroidism

Hyperparathyroidism is the hyperactivity of the parathyroid glands that results in overproduction of parathyroid hormone (PTH). This hormone regulates and maintains calcium and phospate levels. Raised PTH levels negatively affect the bones by causing osteoporosis. High calcium levels in the blood are evidence that calcium is being pulled from the bones.

Calcium is absorbed in the duodenum, which is bypassed in Roux-en-Y and biliopancreatic diversion with duodenal switch surgeries.

Blood tests are used to test for hyperparathyroidism.

Hyperparathyroidism is treated by using Vitamin D supplements, along with calcium supplements.

Protein Malnutrition

Many post-bariatric patients do not get enough protein in their diet and can develop protein malnutrition.

If you remove all the water from the human body, about 75% of what is left is protein. This chemical family is found in every structure in the human body. It makes up the enzymes that power chemical reactions within the body and the hemoglobin that carries oxygen in the blood.

The body contains at least 10,000 different proteins. About twenty building blocks called amino acids form the raw material for all proteins. Amino acids are the structural unit of proteins. Amino acids are critical to life and regulate metabolic function. Twenty two amino acids are considered essential for the body to function and thrive, while a number of other non-essential amino acids are used in various body functions.

Because the body does not store amino acids as it does carbohydrates or fats, it needs a daily supply of amino acids to make new proteins and to replace those that are used in cellular function. About half of the amino acids we need each day are made by the body and are called non-essential amino acids (that is, they are not essential in the diet). About nine amino acids are essential amino acids and must be obtained through food.

Because the body does not store proteins like it stores fats or carbohydrates (in the form of glucose), it needs to consume enough protein each day to provide it with a sufficient amount. Bariatric surgeons recommend 50 to 70 grams of protein a day, with males needing slightly more (70 to 80 grams per day). There are no scientific studies completed to date that confirm these figures in the bariatric population; the amounts have been extrapolated from a historical study of the needs of non-bariatric patients who followed low or very low calorie diets. It is probably safe to assume that you will need to have some protein at every meal in order to get the minimum requirements after weight loss surgery.

Protein deficiency impacts the ability of the body to metabolize nutrients and perform cellular functions.

Some patients suffer from vomiting after bariatric surgery and cannot ingest adequate amounts of protein.

Protein deficiency can result in the excessive loss of muscle mass as the body pulls the proteins it needs from muscle tissue instead of the diet. Most bariatric surgeons prescribe protein supplements to increase the amount of protein, especially immediately after the surgery. Patients might need to continue protein supplementation if their needs are not being met by their post-surgery diet.

Symptoms of protein deficiency include hair loss or brittle hair; loss of muscle mass; wounds that heal slowly or not at all; edema in the hands, feet or abdomen; fatigue; ridges or deep lines in fingernails and toenails; lighter colored hair; skin rashes, dryness or flaking; fainting; and general weakness or lethargy.

Protein deficiency can cause gallstones, arthritis, heart problems, muscle deterioration, organ failure and death.

Protein supplements are available in powder or liquid forms. They are sold in drug stores and health stores or can be ordered online. Because recommended supplemental dosages are high, most people purchase protein supplements in bulk packaging. Some protein supplements intended for weight lifters and sports enthusiasts contain a significant amount of carbohydrates (sugars). Protein supplements intended for bariatric patients contain less sugar. Get into the habit of reading nutritional information panels on any food products you buy.

A common complaint heard after bariatric surgery is that the protein supplements are difficult to drink. I have never found a protein supplement that I would consider tasty. (Some of them can only be described as nasty.) I view protein supplements as another form of medication, and drink it as quickly as I can tolerate it just to get it over with.

Calorie Malabsorption

After bariatric surgery that includes a restrictive component, you will consume fewer calories. In addition, after surgery that is malabsorptive, some of the calories you consume are not absorbed by the body as the food passes through the gastrointestinal tract, as a result of the bypassed section of the intestines. The bypassed section also induces dumping syndrome in Roux-en-Y patients who ingest sugary foods or drinks, in which some calories and significant amounts of fluids are lost.

Calorie malabsorption after bariatric surgery is desirable — this is what promotes the rapid weight loss that patients expect. As time progresses, however, the body adapts to the anatomical changes and begins to process calories in a more optimal way, increasing the amount of calories absorbed from the diet.

For the two year period following your surgery, you will want to maximize weight loss by paying close attention to the caloric intake of the meals you eat each day. After the two year period, it becomes even more important to pay attention to calorie counts.

You must avoid snacking or grazing behavior in which small amounts of food are taken between meals. If you enjoy eating in restaurants, be aware that calorie counts for restaurant foods are usually very high. They can sabotage even people who observe strict portion control or limit snacks.

One area of concern is high-protein drinks. Many bariatric patients become protein deficient and turn to protein drinks to increase the amount of protein in the diet. Be aware of a tendency to consume too many protein drinks; they usually contain significant calorie counts as well as the protein. Eat a varied diet. Protein is available from many sources, so don't rely on protein drinks to get enough of it.

Many obese people have eating disorders. One manifestation is post-surgical eating avoidance disorder (PSEAD), the sensation that after surgery, you will not be able to get enough food to sustain life, or that anything you eat will cause weight regain. If you follow the bariatric diet plan provided by your bariatric surgeon, you'll have no problem with either the quantity or quality of your post-surgical diet.

Some calorie limitation requires lifestyle changes. If you routinely join a group of friends for pizza every week, you might need to find another place to gather with them, like a restaurant that features a salad bar instead, or avoiding restaurants completely and going to a movie. If you can't go bowling without having a milkshake and a large portion of fries, find another hobby. The world is full of people and every one of them has many interests. Finding new friends with new or healthier interests doesn't mean that you'll lose your old friends, it simply means that you can eliminate one more reason for failure.

Anemia

Vitamin B12 deficiency occurs in about 30% of all malabsorptive bariatric surgeries, and about 50% of those who develop a deficiency will develop anemia. Anemia in bariatric patients is also caused by iron deficiency.

For most patients, it is necessary to take iron supplements immediately following surgery and to maintain this practice for life. Many people also require frequent vitamin B12 supplementation, often monthly. Tablets of B12 taken orally are usually not very effective. Bariatric patients should take sublingual or liquid forms of the vitamin, or get B12 injections from their physician.

Anemia is usually preventable and relatively easy to treat.

Achlorhydia

After bariatric surgery, the number of acid-producing cells in the remaining portion of the stomach increases. Many physicians prescribe acid-lowering medication after surgery to control acid levels. These medications then cause a condition called *achlorhydia*, which is characterized by not having enough acid in the stomach to process the incoming food. The food is not digested properly, and patients can develop an overgrowth of bacteria in the gastrointestinal tract. A simple hydrogen breath test can be used to discover if this bacterial condition exists. The overgrowth of bacteria induces nausea and vomiting. Recurring nausea and vomiting changes the absorbency rate of food, which contributes to the vitamin and nutritional deficiencies common in post-bariatric surgical patients.

If you develop achlorhydia, your physician can adjust your medication levels to allow more acid production.

Osteoporosis

Calcium deficiency in post-bariatric surgery patients can cause weakening of the bone that can lead to osteoporosis.

Calcium is absorbed in the duodenum, the upper section of the small intestine that is bypassed after Roux-en-Y and biliopancreatic diversion with duodenal switch surgeries. Calcium deficiencies can cause hyperthyroidism, which causes the parathyroid glands to produce excess parathyroid hormone (PTH). Elevated PTH levels cause calcium to be extracted from the bones, resulting in osteoporosis.

For more information, see "Calcium" on page 157.

Alcohol Metabolism

Post-surgical patients absorb alcohol at a faster rate than people whose anatomy is unaltered, and it also takes longer for the effects of alcohol to wear off. People who have had Roux-en-Y or biliopancreatic diversion with duodenal switch surgeries do not tolerate alcohol well.

You were probably advised to give up alcoholic beverages before your surgery, since consuming alcohol can contribute to some unpleasant side effects during surgery. While you will be able to have an occasional smaller portion of an alcoholic drink in the future, it must be done in moderation.

Some bariatric surgeons will not perform any weight loss surgery on people who have alcohol problems, because it significantly contributes to post-surgical complications.

Issues with Roux-en-Y or Biliopancreatic Diversion with Duodenal Switch

Problems specific to Roux-en-Y or biliopancreatic diversion with duodenal switch surgeries are caused by the process of disconnecting the stomach and intestinal tract and then subsequently reattaching them. Anastomotic leakage usually develops shortly after surgery; for more information, see "Anastomotic Leaks" on page 124. Anastomotic strictures develop over time as the body heals. Anastomic ulcers can be dangerous;

know the symptoms for ulcers and act immediately if you think you have one.

Anastomotic Stricture

The anastomotic connection between stomach and bowel or between two sections of the bowel heals as the body produces scar tissue. Scar tissue tends to constrict over time, which makes the opening smaller. The reduction in the size of the connection is called a stricture.

As food passes through the anastomosis, it stretches it slightly and keeps it open. If the scar tissue becomes inflamed or if the anastomosis isn't stretched enough, the excessive scar tissue can make the opening so small that food cannot pass through it. In the worst cases, even liquids can be obstructed.

Symptoms include pain in the vicinity of the anastomosis. If the anastomosis is significantly blocked, you will vomit whatever food is eaten.

An gastroendoscopic procedure is used to insert a small balloon into the anastomosis. The balloon is inflated and is used to stretch the opening and then removed. The procedure might have to be performed several times to be effective.

Anastomotic Ulcers

Ulceration of the anastomosis occurs in up to 15% of Roux-en-Y and biliopancreatic diversion with duodenal switch patients.

Ulcers can be caused by:

✓ a pre-existing ulcer at or near the surgical site
✓ a restriction in blood supply to the anastomosis in relation to the rest of the stomach
✓ excessive tension on the anastomosis
✓ excess gastric acid
✓ bacterial infection (specifically *helicobacter pylori*)
✓ use of non-steroidal anti-inflammatory drugs (NSAIDs)
✓ smoking

Treatments include:

✓ use of proton pump-inhibiting medications

✓ use of cytoprotectant medications, which increase mucus production in the stomach

✓ temporarily restricting the consumption of solid foods

Ulcers are a serious problem and must be treated. An untreated ulcer can perforate and allow leakage of the contents of the stomach or intestine into the abdominal cavity where it can become infected, cause abscesses, or develop into peritonitis.

As an ulcer develops, it can involve nearby blood vessels and begin to bleed. Bleeding ulcers are significant medically and patients must often be hospitalized for treatment. The presence of blackened stools can indicate a bleeding ulcer for which you should immediately seek medical attention.

Issues with Gastric Bands

Some issues are seen with gastric band surgeries and are caused by the band itself.

Gastric Band Erosion

The gastric band can slowly migrate through the stomach wall to the inside. This can result in symptoms similar to gastritis, but can also be relatively painless. If the eroded area of the stomach is bleeding or leaks the contents of the stomach into the abdominal cavity, surgical treatment is urgently required.

Gastric Band Slippage

While the vast majority of gastric bands remain correctly placed, on rare occasions part of the stomach can prolapse over the band into the restricted pouch area where it does not belong. The enlarged stomach pouch can hold too much food, causing an obstruction that must be surgically repaired. Gastric band slippage is extremely rare.

Malpositioning of the Gastric Band

If the gastric band was not positioned correctly during surgery, no stomach pouch is created. In this case, food intake is limited only if it is too large when it is swallowed; in such cases, the large lump of food cannot pass through the band at all. If the band was not positioned correctly, a revision surgery is performed to correctly place the band, or to remove it completely.

Problems with the Gastric Band Port

The port can move internally so that the membrane cannot be accessed with a syringe from the outside; movement of the port is often accompanied by a kink that develops in the connecting tube. In this case, a minor surgical procedure under local anesthesia is used to reposition the port and remove the kink in the tube. More rarely, the port can be disconnected completely from the tube, or the tube can be punctured during a saline fill attempt, which allows the saline to drain from the band and losing the restriction. Since the saline contained in the band device is sterile, infection is not usually a concern. A minor surgical procedure is performed to replace the port or tube.

Pain at the port site can also be a problem.

12

Vitamin and Mineral Deficiencies

Vitamins and minerals are normally obtained through the foods we eat. They are essential for maintaining life, but most people do not understand why we need them.

Your body requires the appropriate amounts of the necessary vitamins and minerals to function well. In addition to maintaining your health, vitamins and minerals are essential for achieving weight loss goals.

Vitamins regulate the body's core processes, including:

✓ appetite and hunger

✓ brain activity

✓ absorption of vital nutrients

✓ metabolic rate

✓ metabolism of fats and sugars

✓ thyroid and adrenal function

✓ energy storage

No man-made vitamin pill is nearly as effective as getting your daily vitamin and mineral requirements in your diet. However, if your body cannot get the nutrients it needs from your diet, vitamin and mineral supplements can help offset the deficiencies in the diet.

You will need to take vitamin and mineral supplements because:

✓ Malabsorptive surgical procedures reduce your body's ability to absorb vitamins and minerals.

✓ Your smaller stomach cannot hold enough food to supply the quantity of vitamins and minerals you need.

✓ Some bariatric procedures can cause intolerance to foods that contain essential nutrients.

It has been estimated that as much as 80% of bariatric patients are vitamin and mineral deficient before their surgery, making the post-surgical bariatric diet and vitamin and mineral supplementation much more important. Maintaining a sufficient supply of vitamins and minerals helps to ensure your health, helps you lose weight, and helps you maintain your lower goal weight.

	Duodenal Switch	Laparoscopic Gastric Bypass	Adjustable Gastric Band (Lap Band)	Gastric Sleeve	Vertical Banded Gastroplexy
Type of surgery	Malabsorptive	Malabsorptive	Restrictive	Restrictive	Restrictive
Thiamine (B1)	X	X	X	X	X
Folate (B9)	X	X	X	X	X
Iron	O	O			
Calcium	X	X			
Protein	X	X			
Vitamin A	O	X	X	X	X
Vitamin B12	X	O			
Vitamin D	O	X			
Vitamin E	X	X			
Vitamin K	O	X			
Zinc	X	X			
O = deficiency is especially common X = deficiency possible				**Note**: see footnotes 1, 2, and 3 at end of chapter	

Vitamin and Mineral Deficiencies

Ignoring the guidelines for vitamin and mineral supplements can cause medical problems, including death.

Vitamin / Mineral	Deficiency can cause:
Calcium	Bone weakening, brittle bones and osteoporosis.
Iron	Anemia, hair loss and feelings of fatigue.
Folate (Vitamin B9)	Contributes to anemia.
Protein	Most of your major organs are composed of proteins. Deficiencies lead to a number of problems, including muscle deterioration, organ failure, gallstones and death.
Thiamin (Vitamin B1)	Affects the heart, digestive system and nervous system. If deficiencies are not diagnosed and corrected quickly, learning and memory are permanently affected. Can lead to coma and death.
Vitamin A	Can cause night blindness and increases the risk of disease and death from severe infections. If you become pregnant after weight loss surgery, deficiency increases the risk of night blindness and infant mortality
Vitamin B12	Can cause fatigue and tingling in the hands and feet. Can eventually lead to anemia and neurological disorders.
Vitamin D	Can lead to liver and kidney disorders and bone softening diseases.
Vitamin E	Can cause neurological problems, anemia and slow wound healing.
Vitamin K	Increases the risk of osteoporosis and heart disease, increases bruising.
Zinc	Can cause brittle nails and hair loss.

Regular blood tests are required to monitor for vitamin and mineral deficiencies. Displaying physical symptoms is often not conclusive for diagnosis.

You absolutely must commit to taking the correct supplements, in the correct (bariatric) quantity, for the rest of your life. It is not an option to ignore these needs.

Bariatric patients require more supplementation than people who have not had weight loss surgery. The daily minimum requirements chart prepared by the Food and Nutrition Board of the American Institute of Medicine shows the required dietary allowance (RDA) for the **non-bariatric** population. Your bariatric surgeon can provide the appropriate recommended allowances for bariatric patients.

Ensure that every vitamin and herbal supplement you take is approved first by your bariatric surgeon or primary care doctor. If you think you are developing a vitamin or mineral deficiency, don't self-medicate. See your surgeon for blood tests and follow his advice regarding which supplements you need to take. An overabundance of one nutrient can cause deficiencies in other nutrients. For example, taking folate supplements can mask deficiencies for Vitamin B12.

It is important to purchase high-quality supplements. The vitamin and mineral supplements industry is not as tightly regulated as the prescription drug industry, and quality is a major concern. Taking cheap supplements that are inadequate is worse than not taking any supplements at all: not only will you become deficient in the future, but you're also throwing money away on a product that is relatively useless. Effective supplements can be expensive. Bite the bullet and consider it a medication cost, as I do, or include it in your grocery budget. Cheap supplements enable you to save some money now, but bariatric patients who take them are guaranteed to end up spending far more on doctor visits and medications to correct the problems that occur in the future.

It is also important to take vitamin and mineral supplements at specific times of the day. Some supplements do not absorb correctly if taken together, such as calcium and iron. These supplements must be taken several hours apart to be effective.

Finally, ask your bariatric surgeon about taking probiotics. Bariatric patients who took probiotics after surgery had fewer gastrointestinal problems, tolerated food better, and experienced increased weight loss.

Vitamin A

Vitamin A is a fat-soluble vitamin that is needed by the retina of the eye. Since it is fat-soluble, an adequate amount of fat must be included in the diet for Vitamin A to be absorbed.

Vitamin A is essential for maintaining retinal health, but it also plays a function in the immune function, bone metabolism, gene transcription, maintaining healthy skin, promoting the activity of antioxidants, and in the blood.

Females need about 700 mg/day, while males need about 900 mg/day. It is important to obtain the correct dose each day but not to overdose. Because the vitamin is fat-soluble, it cannot be easily removed from the body once it is ingested. Levels of Vitamin A can build up and become toxic. High levels of Vitamin A can contribute to osteoporosis and bone fracture. In many cases, Vitamin K is also found to be deficient because excess Vitamin A prevents certain proteins that are dependent on Vitamin K. Vitamin K deficiency can cause issues with abnormal blood clotting.

Vitamin A is found in the diet in carotene-rich foods (foods that are naturally yellow, orange, or red in color).

Most bariatric patients get enough carotene in the diet, but restrict the amount of fat that is ingested. In the case of biliopancreatic diversion with duodenal switch surgeries, absorption of fat is significantly reduced. In any case, Vitamin A supplements are used. Most bariatric patients can get enough Vitamin A by using a good multivitamin tablet daily; those with higher needs can add a Vitamin A supplement.

Vitamin B1 (Thiamin)

Vitamin B1 or Thiamine is a water-soluble B-family vitamin that is involved in many cellular processes. While plants can synthesize thiamine, humans need to obtain it through the diet. Thiamine deficiency is the cause of beriberi, a disease that was widespread throughout the world and involves the breakdown of glucose. The disease has been widely eradicated in the US because many foods are vitamin-enriched, but it is still a serious problem in alcohol abusers who have a poor diet.

The two forms of beriberi are wet beriberi, which affects the cardiovascular system, and dry beriberi, which affects the nervous system. Wet beriberi can cause congestive heart failure. Dry beriberi causes muscle wasting and partial paralysis.

Thiamine supplements are given by injection or taken orally. Results can be seen quickly, often as soon as one day after administering the thiamine.

Bariatric patients should include unrefined cereals and fresh foods like whole grain breads, fresh meat, legumes, green vegetables, fruit and milk. Supplements can also be used to avoid the deficiency.

Vitamin B7 (Biotin)

Vitamin B7 is also known as Biotin or Vitamin H.

Biotin is necessary for cell growth, the production of fatty acids and in the metabolism of fats and amino acids. It is essential in transmitting carbon dioxide from the body. It is also considered useful in maintaining blood sugar levels.

Symptoms of biotin deficiency include hair loss and a characteristic facial dermatitis in the form of a scaly red rash around the eyes, nose and mouth. Some people have a loss of pigment in the hair.

Because biotin is normally supplied sufficiently in the diet, there are no official guidelines for daily supplementation. If your physician determines that you have biotin deficiency, he can prescribe supplements according to individual need.

Vitamin B9 (Folate)

The human body uses folate in a number of body processes, including in its DNA processes. It helps to produce healthy, viable red blood cells and prevent anemia. It helps avoid heart disease, stroke, and cancer. It also contributes to memory and mental agility, schizophrenia, allergies, rheumatoid arthritis, fertility, renal disease, Type 1 diabetes mellitus, macular degeneration, bone health, menopause, infections, and bone loss with Parkinson's Disease.

Folate supplements can mask problems with Vitamin B12 deficiency. If you take folate, you should have regular blood tests to ensure your vitamin B12 levels are sufficient.

Folate is available in the diet in green leafy vegetables. Flour is frequently fortified with folate (folic acid).

Vitamin B12

Vitamin B12 cannot be produced by the body and must be acquired through diet.

Vitamin B12 deficiency occurs in about 30% of all malabsorptive bariatric surgeries, and about 50% of those who develop a deficiency will develop anemia.

Metabolism of vitamin B12 requires the intrinsic factor produced in the stomach in order to be absorbed further along in the gastrointestinal tract.

The *intrinsic factor* is an unidentified enzyme-like substance secreted by the stomach. It is found both in the gastric juice and the gastric mucous membrane.

As it enters the stomach, B12 binds to haptocorrin, a glycoprotein produced in certain cells in the stomach. The complex enters the duodenum, where pancreatic enzymes digest the haptocorrin. Because the intestinal tract is much less acidic than the stomach, the B12 can then bind to the intrinsic factor. The new compound travels to the ileum, where special cells process it. Inside the cells, the B12 dissociates again and binds to another protein, transcobalamin II. This new compound can exit the cells and enter the liver.

Pernicious anemia is an autoimmune disease in which autoantibodies are directed against the intrinsic factor, which leads to intrinsic factor deficiency, malabsorption of vitamin B12 and megaloblastic anemia.

Pernicious anemia is the loss of the ability to absorb vitamin B12; lowered B12 levels in the blood can indicate the onset of this disease and it can be treated before the patient becomes seriously or dangerously anemic.

Megaloblastic anemia results from the destruction of DNA in red blood cells and is characterized by the presence of many large immature and dysfunctional red blood cells. In pernicious anemia, while red blood cell counts are low, the cells generally develop correctly and function properly. In megaloblastic anemia, red blood cell counts are low and a significant percentage of the cells that remain do not function correctly.

For bariatric patients, oral B12 supplements are ineffective. This is because the oral supplements require the acidic environment of the stomach in order to be broken down and processed by the body. Sublingual doses of B12 in either pill or liquid form are usually effective in doses of 500mg per day or higher. Some people might require B12 to be administered by intramuscular injection on a schedule determined by their physician, usually once per month. Nasal B12 sprays are also available.

It has been noted that post bariatric surgical patients who take probiotics were able to absorb and utilize higher amounts of vitamin B12 than patients who did not take probiotics.

Vitamin D

Vitamin D deficiencies are seen in patients who had distal Roux-en-Y surgery. People who had proximal Roux-en-Y surgery tend to be less deficient in Vitamin D. The deficiency also is common after biliopancreatic diversion with duodenal switch surgery since only 20% of fats that are consumed are utilized.

Vitamin D is essential for bone growth and bone regeneration. It is also integral to the process of regulating the flow of calcium in the bloodstream and resorption into the kidneys, and in absorbing calcium and phosphorus from food as it passes through the intestines. It is required for maintaining cardiovascular health, and it appears to have a function in ensuring longevity. Continuing research also indicates that Vitamin D is an essential defense against cancer cells.

Vitamin D deficiency can lead to osteomalacia, which is a bone-thinning disorder characterized by muscle weakness and frail bone structure. It can also lead to osteoporosis, in which fragile bones lose their mineral density and become porous. Vitamin D deficiency is also linked to a number of immune system disorders and poor cardiovascular health.

The human body normally gets enough Vitamin D from sunlight. It is also available in cod liver oil, but high dosages of cod liver oil can produce Vitamin A toxicity. If Vitamin D is taken as a supplement, many patients do well on a 10,000 IU dose each day.

Vitamin E

Vitamin E deficiencies are seen in patients who had distal Roux-en-Y surgery. People who had proximal Roux-en-Y surgery tend to be less deficient in Vitamin E. The deficiency also is common after biliopancreatic diversion with duodenal switch surgery since only 20% of fats that are consumed are utilized.

Vitamin H

Vitamin H is also known as Vitamin B7 or Biotin. See "Vitamin B7 (Biotin)" on page 154.

Mineral Deficiencies

Calcium

Calcium is absorbed in the duodenum, the upper section of the small intestine that is bypassed after Roux-en-Y and biliopancreatic diversion with duodenal switch surgeries. Calcium deficiencies can cause hyperthyroidism, which causes the parathyroid glands to produce excess parathyroid hormone (PTH). Elevated PTH levels cause calcium to be extracted from the bones, resulting in osteoporosis. Calcium supplements are often combined with Vitamin D to increase absorption.

The type of calcium supplement that is preferred is calcium citrate, which is most easily absorbed into the blood, or calcium gluconate. Another form of calcium supplement, calcium carbonate, requires the acidic environment of the stomach in order to be absorbed; the stomach is largely bypassed after Roux-en-Y and biliopancreatic diversion with duodenal switch surgery and the amount that can be produced by the smaller stomach pouch is not sufficient to maintain an optimal dose.

The optimal dose of elemental calcium is a 500 mg dose taken three times a day. Taking more than 500 mg is not more effective.

Calcium and iron supplements cannot be taken at the same time. Calcium supplements should be taken at least two hours before or after taking iron.

Iron

Iron is often severely deficient after weight loss surgeries. Females, in particular, need additional iron because of the menstrual process. Iron is normally absorbed in the duodenum, which is bypassed in Roux-en-Y and biliopancreatic diversion with duodenal switch surgeries.

Ferrous sulfate can cause constipation and other problems in the gastrointestinal tract even in normal doses, and bariatric patients require additional dosage beyond what is normal. Ferrous fumerate or gluconate can be used, or one of the chelated forms of iron can be used in its place.

Many physicians advise patients who take ferrous sulfate to also take a stool softener at the same time to prevent constipation.

Since iron requires an acidic environment to be processed and absorbed, it can be taken with Vitamin C.

Do not take iron supplements at the same time as calcium supplements. Allow at least two hours before or after taking iron before taking a calcium supplement.

Patients occasionally develop severe anemia even while taking supplements. These patients often must use parenteral iron instead, which is administered by injection or intravenously.

Selecting Supplements

Bariatric patients should take a multivitamin once a day. You can use bariatric multivitamins or those sold in drug and grocery stores. However, you will also need additional vitamin and mineral supplements as prescribed by your bariatric surgeon or primary care doctor, to be taken along with the multivitamin.

Vitamin and mineral supplements are not cheap, and they are not optional. Recent figures for 2008 indicate:

✓ Supplements for patients who had restrictive procedures, like gastric band, gastric sleeve and vertical banded gastroplasty surgeries, costs between $20 and $35 per month.

✓ Supplements for Roux-en-Y surgery patients costs between $35 and $55 per month.

✓ Supplements for biliopancreatic diversion with duodenal switch surgery patients costs $125 or more per month.

If you had pre-existing vitamin or mineral deficiencies before surgery, you will probably need additional supplementation that is more potent than the doses normally prescribed for bariatric patients.

Rather than using general supplements, the best vitamins are those formulated for use by bariatric surgery patients. For example, vitamin B12 pills are not nearly as effective for bariatric patients as sublingual or liquid forms; in some cases, B12 injections might be indicated.

Try an Internet search for "bariatric vitamins" or "bariatric supplements." Your bariatric surgeon probably also has a list of resources, including sources for bariatric supplements.

Note that you can not simply take a multivitamin each day and be done with it.

1 Guy Slater, Christine Ren, Niccole Siegel, Trudy Williams, Di Barr, Barrie Wolfe, Kevin Dolan and George Fielding, "Serum Fat-Soluble Vitamin Deficiency and Abnormal Calcium Metabolism After Malabsorptive Bariatric Surgery." Journal of Gastrointestinal Surgery, Feb 2004. Vol 8, Num 1.

2 E Aasheim, S Bjorkman, T Savik, M Engstrom, S Hanyold, T Mala, T Olbers, T Behmer, "Vitamin Status After Bariatric Surgery: A Randomized Study of Gastric Bypass and Duodenal Switch." Am Journal of Clin Nutrition, July 2009.

3 Robert Kushner, "Managing Micronutrient Deficiencies in the Bariatric Surgical Patient." Treatment of the Obese Patient, Humana Press, 2007. ISBN 9781588297358.

B

Pregnancy After Bariatric Surgery

Pregnancy and childbirth after bariatric surgery are much safer than they would be if you were obese.

Infertility or difficulty in conception can be related to obesity. Losing excess weight can improve your chances for conceiving and bearing children. Obese men and women are more likely to have fertility problems than non-obese people.

Anovulation, a condition in which the body does not release a viable egg each month as part of the menstrual cycle, is a significant fertility issue for obese women. Obese women who lose as little as 5% of their weight can sometimes reverse this problem.

A study was undertaken in 2009 to determine specifically how anovulation was affected following bariatric surgery.[1, 2]

Ninety-eight of the 195 patients who were studied were considered anovulatory before surgery. Seventy patients of the 98 (71.4%) got back to a normal menstrual cycle following surgery. The 28 patients who remained anovulatory lost less weight than the bariatric surgery patients in which the condition was resolved, suggesting that closer attention

---

1   The Endocrine Society Press Release: "Obesity linked to problems that can cause male infertility." http://www.endo-society.org/media/ENDO-07/research/Obesity-linked-to-problems-that-can-cause-male-infertility.cfm.

2   Mandakini Parihar. "Reviews in Gynaecological Practice." Obesity and infertility. Sept 2003. Vol. 3:3, Pgs 120-126.

to the bariatric diet and increasing exercise to improve weight loss could increase the cured rate even more.

Other studies reported the potential improvement in a woman's ability to conceive and give birth to a healthy child after bariatric surgery.[3] In addition to improvements in anovulation, improvements were also noted in menstrual irregularities and polycystic ovarian syndrome, along with more normal hormone levels, which all contribute to increased fertility.

Pregnancy and Complications of Obesity

Obese pregnant women face higher risks of serious complications, including:[4, 5, 6]

✓ development of gestational diabetes (see note below)

✓ pre-eclampsia

✓ delivery by emergency caesarian section

✓ induction of labor

✓ postpartum hemorrhage

✓ genital tract infection

✓ urinary tract infection

✓ wound infection

✓ birth weight below 90%

✓ intrauterine fetal death

Note: Developing gestational diabetes has been shown to nearly double the child's risk of childhood obesity.[7]

3   M Teitelman, et al. "The Impact of Bariatric Surgery on Menstrual Patterns." Journal Obesity Surgery 0960-8923, Nov 2006. Vol 16, Num 11. Pgs 1457-1463.

4   "Some Pregnancy-related Complications Minimized for Women Who Have Had Weight-loss Surgery." Press Release, Nov 18, 2008. Agency for Healthcare Research and Quality, Rockville, MD. http://www.ahrq.gov/news/press/pr2008/barsurgpr.htm

5   The University of Edinburgh Press Release: "Obesity increases pregnancy complications." July 2009. http://www.ed.ac.uk/news/all-news/pregnancy-220709.

6   N Lopez-Duran. "Maternal Obesity During Pregnancy Increases Risk for ADHD Symptoms." Aug 2009. Child Psychology Research Blog. http://www.child-psych.org/2009/08/maternal-obesity-during-pregnancy-increases-risk-for-adhd.html.

7   Pamela Power Scanlon. "A link between gestational diabetes and childhood obesity is reason for leading a healthy pregnancy." Aug 2009. Family Health Examiner. http://www.examiner.com/x-14665-Family-Health-Examiner~y2009m8d6A-link-between-gestational-diabetes-and-childhood-obesity-is-reason-for-leading-a-healthy-pregnancy.

Obese pregnant women also face additional minor complications, including:

✓ ten times greater risk of developing chest infections

✓ more than twice the risk of suffering headaches and heartburn

✓ more than three times more risk for developing carpal tunnel syndrome

✓ more than three times more risk for suffering symphysis-pubis dysfunction (a condition that affects the pelvic joints)

✓ significantly higher risk of depression

Additionally, babies with spina bifida, heart defects, limb reduction defects and hernia of the diaphragm, among other issues, had mothers who were obese.[8] Research indicates that children of obese mothers have an increased chance of developing an attention deficit disorder (ADHD).[9]

Pregnancy Risks by Bariatric Surgery Type

Nutritional deficiencies are more likely following malabsorptive surgeries as opposed to restrictive procedures. However, a study that evaluated different types of bariatric surgery concluded that there were no serious differences between different surgical procedures.[10]

The surgeries evaluated for the study included gastric band surgery, vertical banded gastroplasty (VBG), and Roux-en-Y surgery. The study found:

✓ Patients who had gastric band surgery had significantly higher body mass indexes before delivery

✓ Gastric band patients had more weight gain during pregnancy than VBG or Roux-en-Y patients

---

8   NJ Sebire, M Jolly, JP Harris, J Wadsworth, M Joffe, RW Beard, L Regan, S Robinson. "Maternal obesity and pregnancy outcome: a study of 287,213 pregnancies in London." Int Journal of Obesity Related Metabolism Disorders. Aug 2001. 25(8):1175-1182.

9   Melinda A. Maggard, Irina Yermilov, Zhaoping Li, Margaret Maglione, Sydne Newberry, Marika Suttorp, Lara Hilton, Heena P. Santry, John M. Morton, Edward H. Livingston, Paul G. Shekelle. "Pregnancy and Fertility Following Bariatric Surgery: A Systematic Review." JAMA. 2008;300(19):2286-2296.

10   E Sheiner, et al. "Pregnancy Outcome in Patients Following Different Types of Bariatric Surgeries." Journal Obesity Surgery, Sept 2009. Vol 19, Num 9. Pgs 1286-1292.

✓ The interval between surgery and pregnancy was shortest for gastric band patients (less than 23 months), followed by VBG patients (more than 42 months), with significantly higher intervals for Roux-en-Y patients (more than 57 months)

Birth weight was highest in Roux-en-Y patients compared to the two restrictive procedures

No significant differences were noted in perinatal mortality rates or low birth rates between the groups.

Pregnancy and Bariatric Surgery

If you become pregnant after bariatric surgery, there are some things you'll need to do differently than you would have done before the surgery. However, pregnancy and childbirth after bariatric surgery are generally much safer than they are for obese women who do not have the surgery.

Pregnancy after weight loss surgery has lower risks for maternal complications, including gestational diabetes, high blood pressure and pre-eclampsia. There are fewer premature births, with lower rates for both low and high birth weights.[11]

Two complications of bariatric surgery must be kept in mind: internal hernias and bowel obstruction. The symptoms for these conditions, including pain in the abdomen, swelling or vomiting, resemble normal side effects of pregnancy. If you experience any of these symptoms, consult your physician immediately. Surgery can correct both problems, with good results if acted upon quickly.[12]

Women should avoid pregnancy for the 18 to 24 month period following bariatric surgery. This is the period of greatest weight loss and can be a difficult period for maintaining your body's nutritional needs. You should use the most effective forms of contraception available during this period to prevent pregnancy. Hormonal contraceptives can fail because hormones are no longer absorbed in the correct amount; use barrier contraception instead.

---

11   Agency for Healthcare Research and Quality Press Release: "Some Pregnancy-related Complications Minimized for Women Who Have Had Weight-loss Surgery." Nov 2008. http://www.ahrq.gov/news/press/pr2008/barsurgpr.htm.

12   MS Mirza, et al. "Large bowel obstruction in pregnancy: a rare entity, an unusual cause." Journal Archives of Gynecology and Obstetrics, Feb 2009. Vol 279, Num 2 Pgs 177-178.

Bariatric surgeries that are malabsorptive can prevent the body from absorbing sufficient nutrients. If you plan a pregnancy, or think you might become pregnant after bariatric surgery, you must be careful to take vitamin and mineral supplements. A developing fetus can be harmed by the lack of available nutrients and calories absorbed by the body. Pregnancy during this two year period can also reduce the total amount of weight loss.

Supplements that are especially necessary during pregnancy include:

✓ calcium

✓ iron

✓ vitamin B12

✓ vitamin B9 (folate)

14

My Weight Loss Story

I wasn't always fat. Until I was six, I was rail-thin. Pictures of me at that age show a skeleton with a nice smile.

When I was six, my tonsils constantly caused sore throats, so the decision was made to remove them. This was a very ordinary thing in those days. Every kid had his tonsils out.

After mine came out, I remember having all the ice cream I wanted for a few days, along with dishes of pudding. That was the beginning of the end. I was hooked on sweets and there was no going back.

As a child I had to get my clothes in the Husky Boys section of the stores, while my perfectly-formed younger brother could wear anything off the rack. Well, except for his shoes, which had to be bought in a special store and cost much more than regular shoes. He had enormously wide feet.

I hated having to go to the Husky Boys department, so I ended up only with the ration of new "school clothes" that my mother insisted I have.

I weighed 185 pounds when I graduated from high school. I was chunky but not particularly fat. College was stressful; instead of taking up cigarettes like all of my friends, I located all of the candy bar machines and snacked my way through college years.

I dieted at the drop of a hat. I tried everything. I went to a doctor who prescribed amphetamines. I lost weight and got a hell of a lot accomplished, but it was exhausting, and I regained the weight (plus another ten pounds). I tried all the fad diets. I went to Weight Watchers, Nutrisystem, anything I could find that might work. I always lost weight temporarily but always regained all of what I lost and a bit more each time.

My father died when I was 13, and my mother went back to school to become a nurse. Nursing shifts were long and she worked quite a bit of overtime. I had always enjoyed cooking, working alongside my maternal grandmother, who was an excellent cook, so I started cooking the family meals. There were five of us, so I learned how to cook for five or six people at a time. This proved problematical when I was living alone in later years, since I continued to cook the way I always had: for six people. So I just ate it all. Children were starving in China, my mother told me many times, and I was doing my part.

My worst eating habit developed after I went to work as a secretary at IBM. I was the only male in a completely female profession, and it was stressful. The women didn't know what to make of me, and the men I worked with didn't think I could do the job, even though I had worked as an executive-level secretary for a regional state office previously.

We had 30 minutes for lunch, and at first, my work area was located on the same floor as the best of the three site cafeterias. The food was excellent and cheap and I started eating full three-course meals at lunchtime. Secretaries at that time were assigned to clusters of desks located in the hallways, where everyone congregated, and every secretary's desk had a bowl containing some kind of candy. My desk, of course, had the requisite bowl and I kept it well stocked. Unfortunately, due to my addiction to sweets, I constantly dipped into the bowl too. Before long, I was buying a bag of candy a day and eating most of it myself.

Within two years, I got promoted and went to work as a computer programmer. My office was located in a different area, much farther from the cafeterias, and I started going out to eat at lunchtime. The 30 minute time limit still existed. I learned how to eat quickly, since I had to travel to the restaurant, eat, and return to work all within the 30 minutes.

By the time I reached my mid-30s, my weight was 363 pounds. I developed co-morbid conditions that included heart problems and mild kidney failure. I was also badly injured in two serious car accidents in 1977 and 1993 and suffered a number of broken bones, which made walking difficult.

I began a series of diets in my early 20s that were usually partly successful, but each time I regained more pounds than I had lost. I started to skip breakfast: one less meal a day would help offset the other two. Or so I thought.

In the late 1980s, I went on the Optifast diet (a medically-supervised fasting diet) and was wildly successful. I lost 145 pounds and had to buy an entirely new wardrobe. Activities like walking, biking and even jogging that I had been unable to do before became possible. I enjoy traveling, and after this weight-loss I was able to climb effortlessly to the top of the Tor in Glastonbury, England. The Tor is a steep hillock outside town that has the remnants of an ancient church spire at its peak. Glastonbury is a mystical place, filled with powerful forces, and the top of the Tor is perhaps one of the best known. On this occasion, I was able to easily climb to the top without getting winded or having to make my routine recuperative stop at the bench placed halfway up the path. And when I went back down the steep path, I ran the entire way. The friends who were with me were still near the top while I stood happily at the level of the ring road surrounding the bottom of the Tor, watching them descend. It was the first time I had run in more than twenty years and it felt great!

I was left with a lot of extra skin after this weight-loss. About the same time, I discovered herniated blood vessels in the fat layer of my abdomen that needed to be corrected. I went to a plastic surgeon instead of a vascular surgeon, and he was able to do an abdominoplasty (tummy tuck) at the same time that he did the blood vessel surgery. After 11 pounds of excess skin and fat were removed, I had a waist, a slender profile, and I looked much better than before.

While I was able to maintain this weight loss for several years, I notice my weight begin to creep back upward when my job became very stressful. I fixed the problem with the job by leaving IBM and opening my own technical writing business. It was harder, however, to diet away the extra pounds I was putting back on.

As my heart condition worsened and new problems developed, all of my physicians began to tell me that my lifespan was limited if I stayed as heavy as I was. I ignored their advice for several years. Finally, my cardiologist told me I needed to have a pacemaker installed. I had also become an insulin-dependent diabetic. While I got used to giving myself injections it was never pleasant, and I was not able to eat some of the foods I enjoyed before I became a diabetic.

In 2006, I finally started to research bariatric surgery to see if it was a viable option for me. I decided the best procedure for me was a biliopancreatic diversion with duodenal switch and began looking for a surgeon who could perform that procedure laparoscopically. At that time I lived in Raleigh, North Carolina. Only one local surgeon was performing bariatric surgery of any type, and he only did gastric bypass (Roux-en-Y) surgeries. Because of liability issues, only one hospital in the area allowed the procedures to be done in their surgical center.

I traveled to Atlanta to see Dr Dennis Smith, who performed laparoscopic biliopancreatic diversion with duodenal switch surgery. He agreed to do the surgery and then canceled it when I refused to pay to have another battery of tests and medical consultations identical to the ones I had just completed in Raleigh a month before. I searched for the best bariatric doctor in New York City who did biliopancreatic diversion with duodenal switch surgeries. I found Dr Daniel Herron, who was Chief of Laproscopic and Bariatric Surgery at Mt Sinai Hospital in New York, and went to see him. After an hour's discussion, he made me aware that my co-morbid conditions (heart failure, atrial fibrillation and cardiomyopathy) would prevent me from being a good candidate for a biliopancreatic diversion with duodenal switch. Instead, he suggested having Roux-en-Y surgery, which is easier to perform, takes less time and requires less anesthesia.

The same degree of weight loss that I sought from the biliopancreatic diversion with duodenal switch surgery could also be achieved with the Roux-en-Y surgery. Dr Herron pointed out another benefit that I had overlooked: the Roux-en-Y procedures caused dumping syndrome. For someone who is addicted to sweets, this is most definitely a plus.

Since I had been advised to have Roux-en-Y surgery, I went back to the bariatric surgeon in Raleigh so I could recuperate at home instead of incurring the additional expense of having to stay in New York for two to three weeks. Dr Paul Enochs did the procedure in June, 2007.

The surgery itself was painless. I had only minor discomfort on the day following surgery that was easily resolved by taking acetaminophen. I was released from the hospital two days after surgery, having had to stay an extra day because of my heart condition and the need to monitor my progress after surgery. While I will admit that getting into the car to go home after surgery was uncomfortable, it really wasn't painful. Within a few days, I was back to normal activity.

I had been taking Coumadin, a blood thinner, since 1993 for atrial fibrillation. Because this drug can cause bleeding problems during any surgery, my cardiologist advised me to stop taking the drug a week before surgery. Thirteen days after surgery, I was instructed by my cardiologist to start taking coumadin again at the previous dosage. While I felt that a Protime/INR test (which computes blood clotting time) should be done first, I was told it wasn't necessary. I started the coumadin again on July 3, 2007. The next day, July 4th, I suffered a massive gastric bleed and was rushed by ambulance to a hospital where I received 15 pints of packed red blood cells and three or more bags of plasma. I also had to had two endoscopic surgical procedures to stop the bleeding. I was in ICU for three weeks.

Not eating solid foods was not a problem. For about a month after surgery, I was eating only liquid and very soft foods prepared at the hospital, like dietetic ice cream and sugar-free puddings. I was not hungry at all, which was a good thing, since during the final week in ICU the hospital staff brought some "regular" soft foods. I'm sure hospital kitchens can make even prime rib taste awful, but what appeared on my plate was just nasty. I'd lift the steam cover off the plate, smell the food, and put the cover back on. Not eating that food was not a problem. After I went home and could begin to eat food that was intended for human consumption, my intake increased but I still was never hungry. I had to force myself to eat anything and finally just started eating when the clock told me to.

In my case, my excess pounds didn't just fade way. My weight went down quickly at first and then hit a plateau. It stayed there for several months. The bariatric surgeon kept telling me I had to be losing weight if I was following the diet. I was eating almost nothing, surviving mainly on protein shakes and miniscule portions of soft foods.

My heart condition was to blame. While I was losing fat, I was retaining excess fluid. By the time this was diagnosed I had retained about 60 pounds of excess fluid. It was a long and slow process to reduce the excess fluid, but I began to lose weight again.

It is now 3 years since I had my surgery. My weight remains at a low level, the lowest it's been since high school. I had gotten down to 190 pounds, but looking in the mirror, I looked gaunt and skeletal. I regained about 10 pounds and I think it's improved how I look.

I'm never hungry. I now eat infrequently because I need to eat, not constantly because I want to eat. I recall fearing immediately after surgery that I would not be able to get enough to eat (a condition known as post surgery eating avoidance disorder, or starvation syndrome).

My addiction to sweets is gone. Although I enjoy something with sugar once in a while, I don't gorge on it like I used to. In fact, I generally throw more than half of any sweets away. I never crave sweets like I used to.

While I had been taking supplements during the first year and a half after surgery, I discontinued several of them. I knew I needed them, but life gets busy and frequently, many post-bariatric patients forget having had surgery and begin to concentrate on their new life. I just forgot to buy them. (It's true, my memory is not what it used to be. I have to write down what I had for lunch if I want to remember it that evening.)

From the first day, protein shakes made me nauseous. I eat protein with every meal. I recently became anemic, and realize the value of taking the supplements. As I mention in this book, taking vitamin and mineral supplements is not optional. Your health will suffer, as mine did, if you don't pay attention to your nutrition.

Much of what I've written in this book about life after gastric bypass is based on my own experiences. I have some friends who had weight loss surgeries of various types, and they've been helpful with sharing their own stories as I researched this book.

One friend had a laparoscopic biliopancreatic diversion with duodenal switch surgery. Her surgery was performed the year before mine by a bariatric surgeon in Brazil. She achieved excellent results, and had some difficulties. She pointed out that how people see themselves and how others see them are different after weight loss surgery. People often change a lot of things in their lives, both good and bad. She changed jobs and contemplated leaving her husband. It annoys her when people act as if she should have lost more weight than she did, and people often treat her better than before, which she says also pisses her off. However, I think she is very pleased with her new active life as a thinner person!

Believe me when I say bariatric surgery is a **tool**. It is a pathway into a new life. It is not a quick resolution to a long-standing problem, and it requires commitment and work on your part. I've always said that you can lose the fat, but it knows where to find you.

I wrote this book because when I had my bariatric surgery there was no information, either in books or online, about what to expect after the surgery, other than the weight-loss aspect and a few words about resolving co-morbid conditions. Bariatric surgery involves so much more than that.

It is not an event: it is a lifestyle and a journey.

You will learn that relationships change, your diet changes, even the way you physically eat changes. Not all of the changes are easy to accomplish. Most overweight people are aware that the rest of the world looks at them as defective: something must be wrong with people who can't control their own weight. Yet every overweight person has spent a lifetime trying to lose the excess weight. Many are successful. Unfortunately, success can be fleeting; losing weight can be easy, but maintaining weight loss is difficult unless you make a number of other necessary changes at the same time.

I wish I had a book like this before my surgery. While I still would have had the surgery — I have absolutely no regret about that — I would have had a better idea of what my life would be like as a "thinner person." I would have been more aware that the massive weight loss I saw was only a beginning: maintaining it requires significant commitment and major lifestyle changes.

After bariatric surgery, your life will be a new adventure. Every day will bring changes, some that you like and some you don't like. If you're reading this book, it is likely that you either had weight-loss surgery, or are well along the path of having the procedure. The surgery is the most important thing you'll ever do for yourself. Use this book as a guide to the pitfalls that lie ahead, and a signpost towards success.

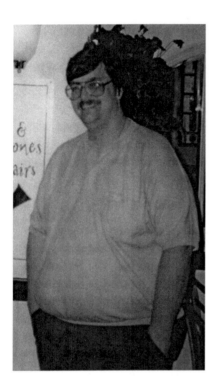

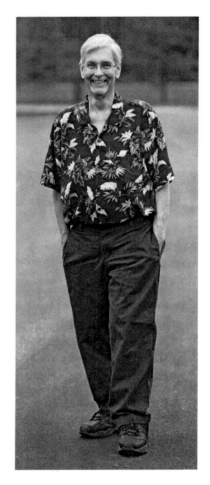

*The author before (left) and
3 years after (right) weight loss surgery*

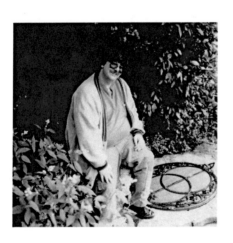

Hints, Tips and Personal Observations

✓ Your grocery bill will not be less because you eat less. Foods that are high in calories, fats and carbohydrates are cheaper than foods that are healthier. My food expenses went up because I now eat healthier foods, mostly fresh or natural products, but because I eat less, it more or less evens out.

✓ Do your weekly grocery shopping by shopping along the outside edges of the grocery store. That's where you'll find fresh vegetables and fruit, fresh meat and seafood, and dairy products.

✓ Be aware of the amount of salt in the foods you eat. Salty foods taste better to most people. Too much salt causes you to retain fluids, and if you have heart issues — not uncommon in weight loss surgery patients — salt exacerbates the problem.

✓ You'll have to buy an entirely new wardrobe. For most people, it's a wonderful thing to finally be able to fit into smaller clothes. After so many years of never looking good in anything, I hate shopping for clothes, and doing it is stressful. However, the joy of being able to walk into any store and buy my clothing from an ample selection right off the rack is incredible. I no longer have to go to special "fat guy stores" and pay inflated prices.

✓ Many, if not most, of your relationships are going to change. It takes time for people to view you in a new light. Give them the time and space they need to do this. Some people will never come around; expect this and let them go. Nature abhors a void; someone new will soon fill the empty spot.

✓ You do not need to turn into an exercise fanatic. You simply need to move your body more than you did in the past. Walking is great; you can do it anywhere, including indoors if the weather is unpleasant, and you can usually talk just about anybody into walking with you. You can enjoy hobbies like bowling, dancing or skating that might have been difficult or impossible before your surgery.

✓ If you were involved with a sport or hobby in the past, resurrect that interest. Overweight people often abandon enjoyable pursuits when the activity becomes uncomfortable for them, and they tend to isolate themselves from social situations in general.

- ✓ If you find yourself snacking (especially at night), you know you are not hungry. If the type of surgery you had created a smaller stomach pouch, you are not likely to be hungry at any point. What feels like hunger can be emotional eating: ingesting food as a defense mechanism to avoid feeling. Stop and ask yourself why you are eating that food at that moment? It is likely that you are eating emotionally.

- ✓ You only have to worry about one day at a time. If you want to lose an extra pound, do it now, **today**, not tomorrow or next week. If you are still losing weight, don't worry about what you'll weigh next week or next year. Concentrate on getting through today. If you feel like eating foods you know you should not eat, or going on a binge, you only have to resist it right now. Find something to do, or go for a walk. Many people eat absentmindedly while reading or watching television; if you do this, be aware of it and do not have food items available when you do these activities.

15

Additional Resources

You can search the Internet to discover a considerable amount of information on bariatric topics. Not everything stated on a website is true, so take the information with a grain of salt and ask your bariatric surgeon about the topic at your next visit. If you do not have access to the Internet, you can visit a public library and ask the librarian for help. Libraries can often request specific reference works from other libraries, so your choices are not limited only to what is shelved locally.

Studies published in book or magazine form referenced in footnotes in this book can sometimes be obtained through your local library system, or at a college or university reference library, or directly from the publishers.

Here are some resources that I found helpful.

Organizations and Websites

✓ American Society for Metabolic and Bariatric Surgery, 100 SW 75th Street, Suite 201, Gainesville, FL 32607. Telephone (352) 331-4900. Fax (352) 331-4875. E-mail: info@asmbs.org.
  http://www.asmbs.org

✓ American Society for Bariatric Physicians (ASBP), 2821 S Parker Rd, Suite 625, Aurora, CO 80014. Telephone (303) 770-2526.
  http://www.asbp.org

✓ Obesity Help website (for weight loss surgery patients).
  http://www.obesityhelp.com

✓ Mayo Clinic website (for general health topics).
  http://www.mayoclinic.com

Diet and Eating

✓ Bariatric Eating website: advice about bariatric diet and nutrition; sells supplements.
  http://www.bariatriceating.com

✓ Bariatric Choice website: advice about bariatric diet; sells foods and supplements.
  http://www.bariatricchoice.com

✓ Bariatric Surgery Nutritional Guidelines from the American Society of Metabolic and Bariatric Surgery (ASMBA).
  http://www.asmbs.org/Newsite07/resources/bgs_final.pdf

✓ Nutritional Eating Disorders Coalition, 603 Stewart Street, Suite 803, Seattle, WA 98101. Telephone (206) 382-3587
  http://www.edap.org

✓ Building Blocks Bariatric Supplements, 4800 NE 20th Terrace, Suite 303, Fort Lauderdale, FL 33308
  http://www.bbvitamins.com

✓ Bariatric Advantage: bariatric supplements
  http://www.bariatricadvantage.com

✓ New Life Bariatric Supplements
  `http://www.newlifebariatricsupplements.com`

Plastic Surgery

Bariatric Plastic Surgery: A Guide to Cosmetic Surgery After Weight Loss. Thomas B. McNemar MD, John LoMonaco MD, and Mitchel D. Krieger MD. Addicus Books, September 2008. 160 pages. ISBN: 978-1886039926.

Total Body Lift: Reshaping The Breasts, Chest, Arms, Thighs, Hips, Back, Waist, Abdomen And Knees After Weight Loss, Aging And Pregnancies. Dennis J. Hurwitz, MD. MD Press, May 2005. 192 pages. ISBN: 978-0974899718.

Body Contouring Surgery After Weight Loss. Jeffrey L. Sebastian, Joseph F. Capella MD, and Peter Rubin MD. Addicus Books, April 2006. 180 pages. ISBN: 978-1886039186.

Bariatric Lifestyle

✓ WLS (Weight Loss Success) Lifestyles Magazine
  `http://store.wlslifestyles.com`

✓ Bariatric TV
  `http://www.BariatricTV.com`

✓ Bariatric Choice website: 12-point exercise plan
  `http://www.bariatricchoice.com/exercise-for-bariatric-gastric-bypass-surgery-patients.aspx`

Finding footnote web references quoted in this book (PMIDs)

References to PMID in footnotes are pointers to specific articles in the PubMed website, which is maintained by the National Institutes of Health. You can determine the correct address on the world wide web by typing the uniform resource locator (URL) this way:

`http://www.ncbi.nlm.nih.gov/pubmed/PMID_#`

where PMID_# is the PMID number shown in the footnote.

For example, to resolve a footnote for PMID 2284209, enter this URL in your web browser, along with the PMID number in the footnote:

```
http://www.ncbi.nlm.nih.gov/pubmed/2284209
```

Footnotes for references that were published on the world wide web might indicate a different URL, which will also display the same article or study as the URL referenced in the PMID.

Index

A

abdominal noises 131
  reducing 131
abdominal pain 65, 138
abdominoplasty 100, 109. *See*
    also panniculectomy
  definition 101
ABMS. *See* American Board of
    Medical Specialties
abscesses 117
absorption rate 53
achlorhydia 143, 146
activated charcoal 137
activity plan 69. *See also* exercise
adhesions 133
adjustable gastric band 8
  and fertility 87
  and insulin 11
  definition 9
  history 7
  illustration of 9
  moderate or no weight loss 11
  productive burping 10
  revision 11
  weight loss compared with
      other surgeries 12
adjustable procedure 10
alcohol 2, 55, 59, 64, 93, 144
alcohol metabolism 144
alimentary hypoglycemia 132
allergic reactions 116
amazon.com 61
American Board of Medical Special-
    ties 94
American Board of Plastic Surgery
    94
American Society of Metabolic and
    Bariatric Surgery 62

amino acids 140
anabolic steroids 93
anagen effluvium 125
anastomosis
  altering to prevent weight gain 56
  and weight gain 57
  complications after surgery 120
anastomotic stricture
  definition 145
  symptoms 145
anastomotic ulcers 145
  treatment 146
anemia 15, 143
  and vitamin B12 143, 155
  iron deficiency 158
anesthesia 94, 97, 98
  complications from 115
  reactions to 115
  twilight 115
anovulation
  definition 161
  in obese women 161
arm lift 100
  definition 101
arthritis 120, 141
ASMBA. *See* American Society
    of Metabolic and Bariatric
    Surgery
aspirin 93
asthma 37
asymmetry 117
attention deficit disorder 163
augmentation surgery
  definition 102
autologous blood transfusion 116

B

back discomfort 99

back lift 100
  bra line 105
  definition 105
bacteria 143
bacterial infection 145
bariatric cooking 60
bariatric eating
  problems 64
bariatric lifestyle
  resources 179
bariatric meals 60
bariatric supplements
  needs after bariatric surgery 152
bariatric surgery 1. *See also* weight loss
  surgery
Bariatric Surgery Nutritional Guidelines 62. *See also* ASMBA
Bariatric TV 79
baseline for weight loss 50
belt lipectomy
  definition 109
beriberi 153
bicep augmentation
  definition 102
bile salts 130
biliopancreatic diversion 8
  history 6
biliopancreatic diversion with duodenal switch 8
  advantages 22
  anastomotic stricture 145
  anastomotic ulcers 145
  and calcium 140, 157
  and flatulence 137
  and iron 157
  and pregnancy 87
  annual blood testing 23
  calcium deficiency after 144
  constipation 128
  definition 20
  diabetes 22
  diarrhea after 134
  diet 21, 22
  disadvantages 23
  estimated cost of supplements 158
  food intolerance 22
  gallstones 23
  history 6
  illustration 21
  issues after surgery 144
  laparoscopic vs open 21
  malnutrition after 23
  nutritional deficiencies 59
  reduction in co-morbidities 22
  revision rate 21
  stomach pouch 23
  ulcers 22, 23
  Vitamin A deficiency 23
  vitamin D deficiency 156
  weight gain 53
  weight loss 50, 53
  weight loss success rate 22
binge eating 40, 51
binge eating disorders 39
biotin 127, 128, 154
  deficiency
    symptoms 154
  needed by human body 154
birth weight 162
bleeding 115, 121
bleeding disorders 116
bloating 65, 135, 138
  swallowing excess air 136
blood
  clots 120, 122
  plasma 116
  tests 151
    for nutritional deficiency 151
  thinners 93
  transfusions 116
blue plate special 68
BMI. *See* body mass index (BMI)
body contouring 100
body image 86
body lift 98
body mass index (BMI) 4

adjustable gastric band 10
  and plastic surgery 93
  definition 4
  determining 4
  higher BMI and complica-
    tion rate 120
bowel obstruction 133
  complications of pregnancy 164
brachioplasty 101
bra line back lift
  advantages for women 105
  definition 105
bread 64
breast implants 106
breast lift 106
breast reduction 107. *See also* breast
  lift
bruising 116
buddy system
  in support groups 78
buttocks enhancement 103
buttocks lift 103

C

calcium
  and iron supplements 157
  and vitamin D 157
  biliopancreatic diversion with
    duodenal switch 140
  carbonate 157
  citrate 157
  deficiency 144, 151, 157
  gluconate 157
  needed in human body 157
  optimal daily dose 157
  pregnancy supplement 165
  Roux-en-Y 140
calf implants 104
calorie malabsorption
  benefits after bariatric surgery 142
  definition 142
carbohydrates 59, 136
carbonated beverages 64

cardiac complications 116
cardiovascular disease 37, 85
carpal tunnel syndrome 163
chafing 99
changing jobs after bariatric surgery
  81
chelated iron 158
chest infections 163
childbirth
  after weight loss surgery 161
childhood obesity
  with obese mothers 163
choosing a plastic surgeon 94
circumferential excess 109
clothing swap 78
cod liver oil
  and vitamin A toxicity 156
coffee 64
common channel 21
co-morbid conditions 97, 116
  complications after surgery 119
  definition 5
  improvement after weight
    loss surgery 37
complication rates 10
complications 94
  bariatric surgery and preg-
    nancy 164
  chances for developing af-
    ter surgery 119
  food addictions 120
  potential after surgery 119
  sleep apnea 120
compression garment 98
concentration, loss of 132
conception
  difficulty in 161
constipation 62, 63, 128
  caffeine and 129
  diuretics and 129
  from iron supplements 158
  stool softeners 129
cookbooks

weight loss 60
coronary disease 97
cramps 65, 138
cravings 66
Crohn's Disease 15

D

death
  and weight loss surgery 37, 141
Decadron 118
deep vein thrombosis 116, 117
deficiencies
  vitamin and mineral 149
degenerative bone disease 38
dehiscence 117
dehydration 96
depression 37, 163
dermatological problems 130
determining medical success after
      bariatric surgery 84
Devrom 137
diabetes 4, 37, 85, 97, 120
diarrhea 7, 22, 62, 63, 134, 138
  biliopancreatic diversion with
      duodenal switch 7
diet 43, 178
  caffeine 48
  meats 47
  planning 66
  resources for 178
  using food journal 66
diet and lifestyle 43
  avoiding fats 47
  changes needed in 44
  chewing food 47
  eating less 46
  eating more slowly 46
  exercise 48
  fluids 47
  fruits and vegetables 47
  hydration 47
  long term changes 45
  meal frequency 46

number of meals 47
  protein 47
  supplements 48
  support groups 48
  sweets 48
difficulty swallowing 62, 63, 123
digestive enzymes 136
dish of the day. See plat du jour
distal Roux-en-Y 18, 156
divorce rate after bariatric surgery 81
drainage tubes 98
dressings 98
drug abuse 55
dumping syndrome 13, 14, 19, 20, 120,
      131
  and blood sugar levels 133
  biliopancreatic diversion with
      duodenal switch 6
  definition 20
  importance of balanced diet 133
  in gastric band surgery 11
  negative aspects 133
  positive aspects 133
  Roux-en-Y 19
  symptoms 132
  vertical sleeve gastrectomy 16
duodenal switch 134
  history 6
dyslipidemia hypercholesterolemia 37
dyspepsia 128
  benefits of 128
dysphagia 123
dysphagia, after gastric band 123

E

early dumping syndrome 132
  symptoms 132
  treatment 133
eating
  resources for 178
eating away from home 66
  and fluids 67
  appetizers 67

avoiding large meals 68
buffets 68
eating at friends' homes 68
food preparation 67
half portions 67
nightclubs 68
portion sizes 67
salad 67
soup 67
splitting portions 67
sports bars 68
eating disorders 39, 65, 142
eating habits
  alternatives to cooking 61
  chewing food 58
  cold foods 58
  daily fluid requirements 58
  drinking fluids 58
  eating away from home 60
  eating while watching TV 59
  fast food restaurants 60
  fluid requirements 58
  fluids, types to avoid 58
  fruits and vegetables 59
  healthy foods 58, 61
  hot foods 58
  irritated stomach 60
  meal frequency 58
  measure foods 59
  minerals 59
  nutritional deficiencies 59
  planning meal times 58
  plate size 59
  protein 58
  reducing starches 59
  skipping breakfast 58
  sugars and fats 58
  supplements 59
  utensil size 59
  vitamins 59
emergency caesarian section 162
emotional eating 65
endoscopy 56

enhancement surgery 100
erectile dysfunction 85
  and co-morbid conditions 85
euglycemic diabetics 18
excess
  abdominal fat 85
  gastric acid 145
  skin 86, 95, 130
    after massive weight loss 89
    and exercise 95
    and slow weight loss 95
    preventing 95
    removing 96
    topical creams for preventing 95
exercise 48, 69
  alternating types to avoid injury 71
  and friends 73
  and loose skin 89
  and obesity 69
  and skin surgery 95
  and weight gain 69
  benefits from 70
  determine body mass index 72
  fitness centers 71
  increasing to prevent
      weight gain 57
  Internet resources 70
  moderate amounts 70
  negative connotation 69
  personal trainers 72
  starting slowly 70
  support groups 73
  walking 70
  with friends 71

F

face lift
  definition 107
fat absorption
  in biliopancreatic diversion with
      duodenal switch 21
fatigue 132
fat necrosis 116

fats 64
  biliopancreatic diversion with
    duodenal switch 7
ferrous
  fumerate 158
  gluconate 158
  sulfate 158
fertility 86
fiber
  insoluble 136
  soluble 136
fibrous foods 64
fixed price meal. *See* prix fixe
flankoplasty 114
flatulence 7, 22, 137
  activated charcoal 137
  biliopancreatic diversion with
    duodenal switch 7, 137
  caused by foods 137
  products to reduce or control 137
  Roux-en-Y 137
flax seed oil 127
fluids
  restrictions on 47
FOG 61
folate
  deficiency 151, 154
  needed by human body 154
  pregnancy supplement 165
follow-up with bariatric surgeon 46
food
  addiction 120
    biliopancreatic diversion with
      duodenal switch 121
    not cured by bariatric surgery 121
  and love 85
  blockage 139
    symptoms 139
    treatment 139
  choices 51
  intolerance
    in biliopancreatic diversion
      with duodenal switch 22

journal 66
  shopping from 66
  tolerance 46
  using to manage stress 85
fried foods 64
fruit juice 64

G

gallbladder disease 4
gallstones 19, 23, 129, 141
  and obesity 130
  bile salts 130
gas 65, 135, 138
  and fats 136
  and proteins 136
  swallowing excess air 136
gastrectomy 15
  illustration 15
gastric acid 145
gastric band
  advantages 11
  disadvantages 12
  erosion 128, 146
  estimated cost of supplements 158
  higher body mass index 164
  insufficient weight loss 57
  issues with 146
  malposition of band 147
  more weight gain dur-
    ing pregnancy 164
  pregnancy risks 164
  problems with port 147
  slippage 146
  tightening, loosening 10
gastric bypass 8. *See also* Roux-en-Y
  definition 17
  history 6
  illustration 17
  weight loss 50
gastric reduction duodenal switch.
    See biliopancreatic diversion
      with duodenal switch
gastric sleeve

estimated cost of supplements 158
gastroesophageal reflux disease 18, 37
  and complication rate after surgery 120
gastroplasty 12
  history 6
  illustration 13
genital tract infection 162
GERD 37
gestational diabetes 162
  lower risks for pregnancy after surgery 164
ghrelin 18, 22
glucose 140
  intolerance 4
goal weight 54
grazing. See snacking
gurgling in abdomen 131
gynecomastia
  definition 110

H

hair loss
  anogen 125
  avoiding 126
  biotin 127
  iron supplements 126
  protein deficiency 127
  telogen 125
  temporary 125
  zinc deficiency 126
haptocorrin 155
headaches 163
health insurance 99
  and staged procedures 9
  approvals from health insurance plan 99
  denial of coverage 99
  plastic surgery procedure coverage 99
  state-level insurance plans 100
  submission to health plan 99

what is covered 99
healthy foods 61
  farm 61
  flavoring 62
  ground 61
  how to prepare 61
  milk products 62
  ocean 61
  replacing fats 62
  replacing oils 62
heart
  defects 116, 163
  problems 141
heartburn 14, 163
helicobacter pylori 145
hematoma 116
hernia 133
  complications of pregnancy 164
  definition 129
  diaphragm 163
  incisional 129
  internal 129
  surgical treatment 129
Hidradenitis Suppurativa 101
high birth rates
  in pregnancy after bariatric surgery 164
high blood lipids 85
high blood pressure 37, 120
  lower risks for pregnancy after surgery 164
high-calorie foods 51
high-protein diet 142
high-risk patients 8
hip lift 114
homeopathic remedies 94
host's table. See table d'hote
hunger 132
hydration 47
hyperlipidemia 4
hyperparathyroidism 140
  and Vitamin D 140
  treatment 140

hypertension 4, 37, 97
hypoglycemia
  alimentary 132
  late dumping syndrome 132

I

IBS. *See also* irritable bowel syndrome
ideal weight 49
implantable gastric simulation 25
implants 103
indigestion 128
  benefits of 128
induction of labor 162
infection 99, 115
infertility 161
insoluble fiber 136
insufficient weight loss 56
intragastric balloon 8, 24
  advantages 24
  definition 23
  disadvantages 24
intrauterine fetal death 162
intrinsic factor 155
iron 157
  and calcium supplements 157
  and stool softeners 158
  and vitamin C 158
  chelated as supplement 158
  deficiency 151, 157
  pregnancy supplement 165
  supplements 126
    and calcium supplements 158
irritable bowel syndrome (IBS) 136

J

jejunoileal bypass 8
  definition 26
  disadvantages 27
  history 5
  pain 27
jejunum 26

L

Lactaid 136, 139
lactose
  digestion 136
  intolerance 138
    Roux-en-Y 138
lap band 8
  definition 9
  illustration 9
late dumping syndrome 132
  symptoms 132
  treatment 133
lifestyle 43
  changes 2
  changes in diet 143
limb reduction birth defects 163
liposuction 92, 108
l-lysine 127
loop bypass 6
loose stools 134
loss of concentration 132
loss of muscle mass 141
love and food 85
low birth rate
  after bariatric surgery 164
lower body lift 108
  and liposuction 109

M

magic pill 2
maintaining goal weight 150
  and vitamins 150
malabsorption 4
malabsorptive bariatric surgery 1, 7
male breast cancer 110
  symptoms 110
male breast reduction
  definition 110
malnutrition 97
malposition of gastric band 147
managing stress 85
mastopexy 106

meal frequency 46
Medicaid 99, 100
  and bariatric surgery 100
  and plastic surgery after bar-
    iatric surgery 100
  what is covered 100
medical issues 86
medical necessity
  plastic surgery 99
Medicare 99, 100
  and bariatric surgery 100
  and plastic surgery after bar-
    iatric surgery 100
medication 93
  changes 95
megaloblastic anemia 155
menstruation 52
metabolic syndrome 37, 38. *See
  also* weight loss surgery
migraines 37
milk products
  reducing intake of 138
minerals
  deficiency 149, 157
    before surgery 150
  deficiency causes 151
  self-medicating 152
mortality rate
  reduction in 2
most popular surgery types 8
muscle deterioration 141

N

National Institutes of Health 4
nausea 65, 116, 118, 138, 139, 143
  after anesthesia 118
neck lift
  definition 112
  vs face lift 108
night eating syndrome 40, 51
nioxin 126
non-alcoholic fatty liver disease 38
non-steroidal anti-inflammatory
  drugs 93, 145
  and gastric band 128
  erosion caused by 128
NSAIDs. *See also* non-steroidal anti-
  inflammatory drugs
nutritional deficiency 59
  achlorhydia 143
nuts 64

O

obesity 1
  and difficulty in conception 161
  attention deficit disorder 163
  birth weight 162
  carpal tunnel syndrome 163
  chest infections 163
  complications from in preg-
    nancy 162
  depression 163
  effects of 33
  emergency caesarian section 162
  genital tract infection 162
  gestational diabetes 162
  headaches 163
  heartburn 163
  heart defects 163
  hernia of diaphragm 163
  induction of labor 162
  intrauterine fetal death 162
  limb reduction birth defects 163
  postpartum hemorrhage 162
  pre-eclampsia 162
  spina bifida 163
  symphysis-pubis dysfunction 163
  urinary tract infection 162
  wound infection 162
Optifast 54
organ failure 141
organizations 178
orthopedic problems 38
osteomalacia 156
osteoporosis 144
outer thigh lift 114

overeating 62

P

pain 65, 116
  after jujunoileal bypass 27
panniculectomy 100. *See also* abdomi-
    noplasty
  definition 113
passing out 132
pasta 64
pectoral implants 104
Pepcid AC 118
pernicious anemia 155
personal trainers 72
  finding 72
  what to avoid 73
pie hole
  and weight gain 54
pitfalls leading to weight gain 54
plastic surgery 89
  alcohol 93
  American Board of Plas-
      tic Surgery 94
  anabolic steroids 93
  anesthesia 97
  arm lift 101
  aspirin 93
  asymmetry 117
  augmentation 102
  autologous blood transfusion 116
  back lift 105
  bargain pricing 97
  bicep augmentation 102
  bleeding disorders 116
  blood
    clotting 93
    thinners 93
    transfusions 116
  BMI 93
  body lift 98
  brachioplasty 101
  bra line back lift 105
  breast

  implant 106
  lift 106
  lift and body lift 107
buttocks
  enhancement 103
  lift 103
calf implants 104
cardiac complications 116
choosing a plastic surgeon 94
choosing the correct type
    of surgeon 96
co-morbid conditions 97, 99
complications 94
  of anesthesia 93
compression garment 98
considerations after plas-
    tic surgery 102
deep vein thrombosis 116, 117
determining which proce-
    dures to have 97
dressings 98
face lift 107
flankoplasty 114
gynocomastia 110
health insurance 99
heart disease 116
Hidradenitis Suppurativa 101
hip lift 114
homeopathic remedies 94
implants 103
lifting restrictions 93
liposuction 108
lower body lift 108
male breast reduction 110
mastopexy 106
medication changes 93, 95
navel placement 117
neck lift 112
non-steroidal anti-inflam-
    matory drugs 93
not an obesity operation 116
nursing care after surgery 98
order of surgical procedures 98

outer thigh lift 114
pain 98, 117
panniculectomy 113
paying for 96
pectoral implants 104
platysmaplasty 112
potential risks 115
pregnancy 93
pulmonary complications 116
realistic expectations 99
recovery 102
recreational drug usage 93
referrals from bariatric surgeon 97
resources for 179
revisional surgery 95
risks like bariatric surgery risks 115
scars 117
scheduling after weight loss 92
side effects from 115
skin sensation 117
smoking 93
spiral thighplasty 114
staged
    procedure 98
    reconstruction 98
thigh lift 114
tricep augmentation 102
using autologous blood
        transfusion 116
vertical thighplasty 114
vitamins 94
when medically necessary 99
wound separations 117
plat du jour 68
platysmaplasty 112
polycystic ovarian syndrome 38
popcorn 64
portion sizes 3, 51, 62
    eating less 62
    weighing food 63
postpartum hemorrhage 162
post surgical eating avoidance disor-
        der 51

potency
    increasing after mas-
        sive weight loss 87
potential complications 119
potential problems 119
pre-eclampsia 162
    lower risks for pregnancy af-
        ter surgery 164
pregnancy
    after bariatric surgery 161
    after weight loss surgery 164
    biliopancreatic diversion with
        duodenal switch 87
    complications of obesity 162
    malabsorptive surgeries 165
    problems in obese women 86
    risks
        by bariatric surgery type 163
        gastric band 164
        Roux-en-Y 164
        vertical banded gastroplasty 164
    Roux-en-Y 87
    time period to avoid after bar-
        iatric surgery 165
premature births
    fewer after weight loss surgery 164
prix fixe 68
probiotics 135
    and supplements 152
    and vitamin B12 absorption 156
problems
    abdominal noises 131
    achlorhydria 143
    anastomotic
        stricture 145
        ulcers 145
    anemia 143
    bleeding 121
    bloating 135
    blood clots 122
    bowel obstruction 133
    carbohydrates 136
    chest pain 65

constipation 128
dermatological 130
diarrhea 134
difficulty swallowing 123
digestive enzymes 136
discomfort 65
dumping syndrome 131
dyspepsia 128
dysphagia 123
early dumping syndrome 132
excess skin 130
feeling cold 131
feeling full 64
flatulence 137
food blockage 139
gallstones 129
gas 135
gastric band
  erosion 146
  malposition 147
  port problems 147
  slippage 146
gurgling in abdomen 131
hernia 129
hyperparathyroidism 140
incisional hernia 129
indigestion 128
internal hernia 129
irritable bowel syndrome 136
lactose
  digestion 136
  intolerance 138
late dumping syndrome 132
long-term 127
loose stools 134
milk products 138
osteoporosis 144
potential after surgery 119
pressure in chest 65
protein malnutrition 140
pulmonary embolism 122
skin 130
staple failure 124

steatorrhea 134
stomal stenosis 139
swallowing excess air 136
telogen effluvium 125
temporary hair loss 125
thrush 127
ulcers 128, 145
with bariatric eating 64
wound infection 122
yeast infection 127
productive burping 10
protein
  amino acids 140
  daily allowance for bariat-
      ric patients 140
  deficiency 127, 151
    loss of muscle mass 141
    problems from 141
    symptoms 141
  in human body 140
  malnutrition 140
  supplements 141
proximal Roux-en-Y 18, 156
PSEAD. *See* post surgical eating
      avoidance disorder
pseudotumor cerebri 38
ptosis
  definition 106
  determining severity of 106
  of breasts in women 106
pulmonary
  complications 116
  embolism 122
pyloric valve 22, 131, 133
  vertical sleeve gastrectomy 16

R

reaction to medications 115
recreational drug usage 93
red meat 64
relationships 81
  and romance 81
  concerns with after bariat-

ric surgery 84
coping 82
how people treat you after
    bariatric surgery 81
improving after bariatric surgery 82
significant others 82
with food 81
with people 81
reoperation 4
resources 177
  bariatric lifestyle 179
  diet 178
  eating 178
  organizations 178
  plastic surgery 179
  published studies 177
  studies quoted in this book 177
  websites 178
restaurants 66
Restorative Obesity Surgery, Endolu-
    minal 56
restrictive bariatric surgery 1, 7
restrictive procedures
  vs malabsorptive procedures 120
reversible
  adjustable gastric band 9
risks 5
ROSE technique 56. *See also* restor-
    ative obesity surgery, endolu-
    minal
Roux-en-Y 6, 8
  addiction to sweets 121
  advantages 18
  anastomotic
    stricture 145
    ulcers 145
  annual blood tests 19
  back pain 19
  birth weight 164
  blood tests 19
  calcium absorption 140
  calcium deficiency 144, 157
  constipation 128

definition 17
diarrhea after 134
disadvantages 19
distal 18, 156
dumping syndrome 19, 20
estimated cost of supplements 158
euglycemic diabetes 18
flatulence 137
gallstones 19
gastroesophageal reflux disease 18
hunger 20
illustration 17
iron 157
issues after surgery 144
laparoscopic, history 7
malabsorption 19
meal plan 20
mortality rates 19
nutritional deficiencies 59
pregnancy 87
pregnancy risks 164
proximal 18, 156
reduction in co-morbidities 18
venous thromboembolic disease 19
vitamin D deficiency 156
weight gain 53
weight loss 50, 53
weight loss success rate 18

S

scars 115
  reducing by using topi-
      cal sterioids 118
sclerosant 56
secret of successful weight loss 48
selecting supplements 158
self-medicating
  vitamins and minerals 152
self-perception after surgery 82
sepsis 120
  complications after surgery 120
seroma 116
set menu 68

sex 85
  no correlation between satisfac-
    tory sex life and obesity 86
  obesity-related problems 85
  unrealistic expectations after
    bariatric surgery 85
sexual health
  link to emotional health
    in women 86
  link to physical health in men 85
shakiness 132
side effects 4
silica 127
silicone implants 104
silicone ring
  to prevent weight gain 56
skin
  problems 130
  sensitivity 117
  surgery 95
    dehydration 96
    exercise 95
    malnutrition after bar-
      iatric surgery 95
    meal plans 96
    preventing 95
sleep apnea 4, 38, 97, 120
  and complications after surgery 120
sleeve gastrectomy 8, 15. See also bil-
    iopancreatic diversion with
    duodenal switch
sleeve gastrectomy with duodenal
    switch 8. See also biliopancre-
    atic diversion with duodenal
    switch
smoking 2, 93, 94, 146
snacking 50
snacks 59
soluble fiber 136
spina bifida 163
spiral thighplasty 114
staged
  procedure 8, 98

health insurance plans 9
  vertical sleeve gastrectomy 15
  reconstruction 98
staple failure 124
starvation syndrome 41, 51. See
    also post surgical eating avoid-
    ance disorder
steatorrhea 134
steroids 93
stomach pouch
  size after restrictive surgery 62
stomach stapling 6
stomal stenosis
  definition 139
stress urinary incontinence 38
sugars 64, 135
supplements 23, 130, 150, 151
  bariatric needs 152
  bariatric quality 152
  cost by bariatric surgery type 158
  for pregnancy
    calcium 165
    folate 165
    iron 165
    vitamin B9 165
    vitamin B12 165
  pregnancy 165
  protein 141
  selecting 158
  taking correct bariatric types 159
  when to take 152
  with pre-existing nutritional
    deficiencies 158
support group 48, 55, 66, 73, 75
  achieving weight loss goals 75
  advantages 75
  and less weight regain 76
  atmosphere 78
  body mass index (BMI) 75
  buddy system 78
  choosing 77
  clothing swap 78
  dealing with problems 75

exposure to weight loss progress 76
family and friends 76
gastric band 75
guest speakers 78
in-person 76, 77
lap band 75
maintaining motivation 76
moderated 77
participating 78
positive attitude 78
positive vs negative tone 78
recipes from 61
referrals to other resources 78
remote 77
size 77
specific for surgery type 77
starting your own 77
virtual 77
virtual - availability 79
virtual participating 79
where to find 76
surgery to prevent weight gain 56
sutures
  problems with 116
swallowing excess air 136
sweating 132
sweets 64
swelling 116
symphysis-pubis disorder 163

T

table d'hote 68
telogen effluvium 125
temporary hair loss 125
thiamin
  deficiency 151
  needed by human body 153
thigh lift 100, 114
thrombosis, deep vein 117
thrush 127, 128
transcobalamin II 155
tricep augmentation 102
trying new foods 63

tummy tuck. *See* abdominoplasty

U

ulcers 22, 23, 128, 145
  gastric band erosion 128
  risk of developing 128
urinary tract infection 162
using smaller plates 63

V

vagotomy 25
vagus nerve 25
venous insufficiency 97
venous stasis disease 38
venous thromboembolic disease 19
vertical banded gastroplasty 8
  advantages 13
  definition 12, 15
  diet restrictions 13
  disadvantages 13
  dumping syndrome 14
  estimated cost of supplements 158
  heartburn 14
  history 6
  illustration 13
  mortality rate 13
  nutritional issues 13
  pregnancy risks 164
  weight regain 14
vertical sleeve gastrectomy 15
  advantages 16
  definition 15
  disadvantages 16
  duodenum 16
  illustration 15
  long term success rate 16
  malabsorption in 16
vertical thighplasty 114
vitamin A
  deficiency 151
  diet 153
  for females 153
  needed by human body 152

toxicity
  and cod liver oil 156
vitamin B1
  and beriberi 153
  deficiency 151
  needed by human body 153
vitamin B7
  deficiency
    symptoms 154
  needed by human body 154
vitamin B9
  deficiency 151, 154
  needed by human body 154
  pregnancy supplement 165
vitamin B12 143
  and intrinsic factor 155
  deficiency 151, 155
  dosage requirements for bar-
    iatric patients 143
  needed by human body 155
  pregnancy supplement 165
  types of supplements to take 155
vitamin C
  and iron 158
vitamin D 140, 156
  and calcium 157
  deficiency 151, 156
    biliopancreatic diversion with
      duodenal switch 156
    Roux-en-Y 156
  needed in human body 156
vitamin E
  deficiency 151, 156
  needed in human body 156
vitamin H. *See* biotin; *See also* vitamin
    B7
  deficiency
    symptoms 154
  needed by human body 154
vitamin K
  deficiency 151
vitamins 94
  and weight loss 150

deficiency 149
  before surgery 150
  deficiency causes 151
  maintaining goal weight 150
  requirements by human body 149
  self-medicating 152
vomiting 62, 63, 65, 118, 139, 141, 143

W

weakness 132
websites 178
weighing daily 54
weight gain 53
  biliopancreatic diversion with
      duodenal switch 53
  minimizing 54
  nutritionist 57
  pitfalls 54
  reversing with surgery 56
  Roux-en-Y 53
  secret for minimizing 54
weight loss 27, 52
  adjustable gastric band 11, 52
  and body image 86
  and vitamins 150
  baseline 50
  biliopancreatic diversion with
      duodenal switch 52, 53
  early 51
  gastric band 52
  gastric bypass 52
  insufficient after surgery 56
  lap band 52
  maximizing 142
  medical issues 86
  objectivity 86
  relative to surgery date 50
  Roux-en-Y 52, 53
  secret for success 49
weight loss surgery 1
  and pregnancy 161
  binge eating disorders 39
  co-morbid conditions 28

estimates of weight loss by
    surgery type 29
myths 31
not reversible 28
WLS 1, 2, 3, 6, 9, 15, 16,
    20, 22, 23, 27
weight plateau
  diet 52
  eating habits 52
  exercise 53
  fluids with meals 53
  menstruation 52
  overcoming 52
what not to eat 63
willpower 3
WLS Lifestyles 79
wound infection 122, 162
wound separations 117

Y

yeast infection 127

Z

zinc
  deficiency 126, 151
  sulfate 126
Zofran 118

CPSIA information can be obtained at www.ICGtesting.com

225030LV00007B/146/P